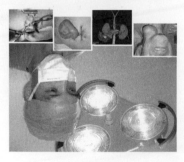

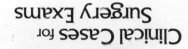

Clinical Cases for Surgery Exams

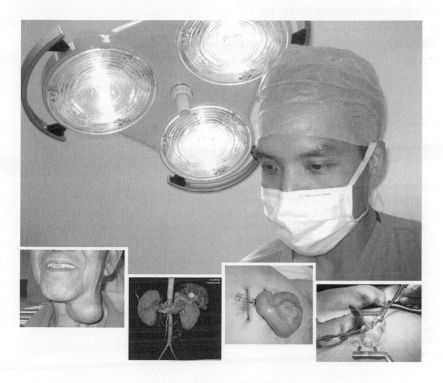

Clinical Cases for
Surgery Exams

Charles T K Tan
National University of Singapore, Singapore

Co-editors

Thiam-Chye Lim • Peter A Robless
National University of Singapore, Singapore

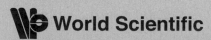 **World Scientific**

NEW JERSEY · LONDON · SINGAPORE · BEIJING · SHANGHAI · HONG KONG · TAIPEI · CHENNAI

Published by

World Scientific Publishing Co. Pte. Ltd.

5 Toh Tuck Link, Singapore 596224

USA office: 27 Warren Street, Suite 401-402, Hackensack, NJ 07601

UK office: 57 Shelton Street, Covent Garden, London WC2H 9HE

Library of Congress Cataloging-in-Publication Data
Lim, Thiam-Chye.
   Clinical cases for surgery exams / Thiam-Chye Lim, Peter A. Robless, Charles T.K. Tan.
      p. ; cm.
   Includes index.
   ISBN-13: 978-981-283-552-9 (pbk. : alk. paper)
   ISBN-10: 981-283-552-0 (pbk. : alk. paper)
   1. Surgery--Examinations, questions, etc. I. Robless, Peter A. II. Tan, Charles T.K. III. Title.
   [DNLM: 1. Diagnosis--Examination Questions. 2. General Surgery--Examination Questions.
3. Pathology, Surgical--Examination Questions. WO 18.2 L732s 2009]
   RD37.2.L56 2009
   617--dc22

                                                                2009009705

British Library Cataloguing-in-Publication Data
A catalogue record for this book is available from the British Library.

Printed by FuIsland Offset Printing (S) Pte Ltd, Singapore

*We dedicate this book
to our families, whose support
made this work possible.*

To my family; Audra, Craig and Claire

Charles

FOREWORD

The Halstedian preceptorship has been the bed rock of surgical training for over a century. While an orderly & graduated clinical experience is desirable, its well known drawbacks have become evident especially in the current environment. There have been significant changes in the methodology of imparting and acquiring clinical knowledge and its assessment and evaluation.

The written "essay" MCQ "long & short" case and the "clinical viva" still has a place in the total evaluation of candidates. Other modalities have come into the fore. The OSCE system has been used for evaluation of knowledge and assessment in the examination setting. Its focus is on a specific clinical problem, illustrated by various means which requires a specific answer. Unless one has the background knowledge (basic sciences and its clinical application) it would be difficult to comprehend and effectively answered the questions posed.

The authors have collected a wide and clinically relevant scenarios for which specific and pertinent questions are asked of the student. It covers most surgical specialties. It cannot replace the surgical text, but it should stimulate the student to "read up" on the clinical problem illustrated from surgical texts, monographs and journals. It is not a short cut to the acquisition of knowledge and understanding of clinical surgery.

The authors are to be congratulated in their effort to cover most aspects of clinical surgery encountered in daily practice. This book should be useful to both under and post-graduate students for revision and reinforcement of a knowledge base and expose them to the OSCE system and a honest self evaluation.

Abu Rauff MB MS FRCS FAMS
Senior Consultant
National University Health System
Adj Professor
Yong Loo Lin School of Medicine

FOREWORD

The teaching of surgery, both at an undergraduate and postgraduate level has been made increasingly difficult in the current era of cost-constrained surgical care and ambulatory surgery. Not so long ago, surgeons could teach their students and surgical residents the entire spectrum of surgical diagnosis and management on ward rounds and in hospital outpatient clinics. Hospitals used to be full of patients displaying the full range of surgical pathology. Nowadays few patients get to spend any time in a hospital bed. Surgical patients are admitted day of surgery, such that wards no longer contain any pre-operative patients with surgical signs suitable for teaching. Likewise early discharge from hospital for most patients having elective surgery has meant that the only inpatient surgical cases are those with major trauma or complex life-threatening disease. The simple hernia is no longer to be seen in a hospital, other than for a fleeting hour or so between the fast-track admission office and the anaesthetic bay. In Australia at least, surgical outpatients have also been largely abolished in most major university teaching hospitals, with the pre-operative assessment and post-operative care of all patients privatised and moved to individual surgeon's office. Even the outpatient clinic has disappeared as a source of teaching material. Thus this book by Tan and his colleagues provides a timely resource for teaching surgery. Whilst clinical bedside teaching can never be completely replaced, this book presents a comprehensive set of short answer questions relevant to surgical candidates at both the undergraduate and postgraduate level. There are a series of chapters which cover the surgical specialties as well as all the subspecialties within general surgery, such as breast, endocrine, upper GI and hepatobiliary. Most importantly the visual cues presented by the clinical photographs accompanying each question provide an invaluable resource for both students and teachers alike. At the end of each chapter, a comprehensive "correct" response is given to each question, allowing immediate feedback and positive reinforcement to the candidate. I am sure this book will prove to be an invaluable resource for surgical teaching.

Leigh Delbridge MD FRACS
Professor of Surgery
University of Sydney

PREFACE

This book is intended for candidates who are taking undergraduate and postgraduate surgical examinations. It is by no means exhaustive but provides valuable visual revision material to reinforce the student's knowledge of the core subjects. The questions are accompanied by pictures and are similar to those which may be asked at a viva examination. Additionally, the book highlights surgical pathology peculiar to the Asian population.

At present, the medical student to patient ratio in Singapore is increasing. There are now more medical students and fewer in-patients in hospital wards to facilitate clerkship and the diagnoses of diseases. More medical examinations are now conducted with computers and photographs of surgical pathology as the recruitment of patients for such examinations become more difficult. This book will be useful in presenting the candidate with the various surgical problems they might encounter in future.

The book is divided into 14 chapters, with questions posed at the front and answers on the back page. This arrangement allows the reader to formulate their own answers beforehand.

This book cannot be used as a replacement for clinical teaching. However, it does aspire to provoke thought amidst diagnostic challenges, aiming to improve the surgical acumen of a surgeon-to-be.

Finally, most of these cases were encountered in the course of our surgical career, and have been archived with the intention for sharing with our medical colleagues.

Enjoy surgery.

Charles T K Tan
Peter A Robless
T C Lim

ACKNOWLEDGEMENTS

A special thanks to all the surgical colleagues, patients and students who have contributed to this book.

CONTENTS

CONTENTS

EDITORS

Charles T K Tan
MBChB, M.Med (Surgery), FRCS(Ed)(Gen Surgery), FAMS
Consultant
Division of Endocrine and Minimally Invasive Surgery
Department of Surgery
National University Health System

CO-EDITORS

Peter A Robless
MBChB, FRCS(Ed)(Gen Surgery), MD, FEBVS
Senior Consultant
Department of Cardiothoracic & Vascular Surgery
National University Health System
Associate Professor
Yong Loo Lin School of Medicine

T C Lim
MBBS, FRCS(Ed), FAMM, FAMS (Plastic Surgery)
Senior Consultant and Head
Division of Plastic, Reconstructive and Aesthetic Surgery
Department of Surgery
National University Health System
Associate Professor
Yong Loo Lin School of Medicine

LIST OF CHAPTER AUTHORS

T C Lim*
MBBS, FRCS(Ed), FAMM, FAMS (Plastic Surgery)
Senior Consultant and Head
Division of Plastic, Reconstructive and Aesthetic Surgery
Department of Surgery
National University Health System
Associate Professor
Yong Loo Lin School of Medicine

Dale L S K Loh
BA, MBChB, FRCS(Paediatric Surgery), FAMS
Consultant
Department of Paediatric Surgery
National University Health System

S Suresh Nathan
MBBS, M.Med(Surgery), FRCS(Ed), FAMS(Ortho)
Consultant
Department of Orthopaedic Surgery
National University Health System
Assistant Professor
Yong Loo Lin School of Medicine

K Prabhakaran
MBBS, FRCS(Ed), FRCS(Glas), FAMS
Senior Consultant & Head
Department of Paediatric Surgery
National University Health System
Associate Professor
Yong Loo Lin School of Medicine

* All chapters by Charles TK Tan, Peter A Robless and TC Lim unless otherwise stated.
** Contributed to pathological aspects of various conditions.

Peter A Robless*
MBChB, FRCS(Ed)(Gen Surgery), MD, FEBVS
Senior Consultant
Department of Cardiothoracic & Vascular Surgery
National University Health System
Associate Professor
Yong Loo Lin School of Medicine

Kong Bing Tan**
MBBS, FRCPath, FRCPA, ICDP-UEMS
Consultant
Department of Pathology
National University Health System
Assistant Professor
Yong Loo Lin School of Medicine

Charles T K Tan*
MBChB, M.Med (Surgery), FRCS(Ed)(Gen Surgery), FAMS
Consultant
Division of Endocrine and Minimally Invasive Surgery
Department of Surgery
National University Health System

LIST OF ABBREVIATIONS

5FU	5 Flourouracil
AAA	Abdominal Aortic Aneurysm
ABPI	Ankle Brachial Pressure Index
AFB	Acid Fast Bacilli
AFP	Alpha Feto Protein
APACHE	Acute Physiology and Chronic Health Evaluation
APC	Adenomatous Polyposis Coli
ARDS	Acute Respiratory Distress Syndrome
ATLS	Advanced Trauma Life Support
AVM	Arteriovenous malformation
BCC	Basal Cell Carcinoma
BCG	Bacillus Calmette-Guerin
BMI	Body Mass Index
BPH	Benign Prostatic Hypertrophy
BRCA	Breast Cancer Gene
CBD	Common Bile Duct
CD117	Cluster of Differentiation 117/ C-kit Receptor
CPP	Cerebral Perfusion Pressure
CSF	Cerebro Spinal Fluid
CT	Computer Tomography
CXR	Chest X Ray
DCIS	Ductal Carcinoma In Situ
DPL	Diagnostic peritoneal lavage
DTPA	Technetium Labelled DiethyleneTriminepentacetic Acid
DVT	Deep Vein Thrombosis
EBV	Epstein Barr Virus
ECG	ElectroCardioGram
EPL	Extensor Pollicis Longus
ER	Estrogen Receptor
ERBB2	v-erb-b2 erythroblastic leukaemia viral oncogene
ERCP	Endoscopic Retrograde CholangioPancreatography

ESR	Erythrocyte Sedimentation rate
ESWL	Extracorporeal Shockwave Lithotripsy
EUA	Examination Under Anaesthesia
EUS	Endoscopic Ultrasound
FAP	Familial Adenomatous Polyposis
FAST	Focussed Abdominal Sonography for Trauma
FHH	Familial Hypocalciuric Hypercalcaemia
FNAC	Fine Needle Aspiration Cytology
FTSG	Full Thickness Skin Graft
GCS	Glasgow Coma Score
GFR	Glomerular Filtration rate
HCC	Hepatocellular carcinoma
HD	Haemodialysis
HIDA	Hepatobiliary Imino-Diacetic Acid scan
HIV	Human Immunodeficiency virus
HNPCC	Hereditary Non Polyposis Colorectal Cancer
HPV	Human Papilloma Virus
ICP	Intracranial Pressure
IJV	Internal Jugular Vein
IPMN	Intraductal Papillary Mucinous Neoplasm
IVC	Inferior Vena Cava
LHRH	Luteinising Hormone-Releasing Hormone
LOS	Lower Oesophageal Sphincter
MEN	Multiple Endocrine Neoplasia
MRA	Magnetic Resonance Angiography
NAC	Nipple-areola Complex
NPC	Nasopharyngeal carcinoma
NSCLC	Non Small Cell Lung Cancer
OCH	Oriental Cholangiohepatitis
OPSI	Overwhelming Post Splenectomy Infection
ORIF	Open Reduction Internal Fixation
PCN	Percutaneous Nephrostomy
PCNL	Percutaneous Nephrolithotripsy
PD	Peritoneal dialysis
PE	Pulmonary Embolism
PEEP	Positive End Expiratory Pressure

PEG	Percutaneous Endoscopic Gastrostomy
PET	Positron Emission Tomography
PPD	Purified protein Derivitive
PPI	Proton pump Inhibitor
PR	Progesterone Receptor
PSA	Prostate Specific Antigen
PTC	Percutaneous Transhepatic Cholangiogram
PTH	Parathyroid Hormone
RPP	Retropubic prostatectomy
SCLC	Small Cell Lung Cancer
SDH	Subdural Haematoma
SSI	Surgical Site Infection
STSG	Split thickness Skin Graft
TEM	Transanal Endoscopic Microsurgery
TIPS	Transjugular Intrahepatic Portalsystemic Shunt
TNM	Classification of Malignant Tumours (TNM) by the International Union against Cancer (UICC)
TPN	Total Parenteral Nutrition
TPO	Thyroid Peroxidase
TSH	Thyroid Stimulating hormone
TURBT	Transurethral Resection Bladder Tumour
TURP	Transurethral Resection Prostate
TVP	Transvesical prostatectomy
VACTERAL	Vertebral Anorectal Cardiac Tracheal Eosphageal Renal and Limbs
VHL	von Hippel Lindau
VMA	Vanillyl Mandelic Acid

Chapter 1

GENERAL SURGICAL PRINCIPLES

Q1.1
This patient had a liver abscess and was in the Intensive Care Unit.

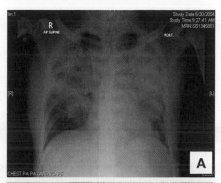

A. What can be seen in the chest X-ray (picture A)?

B. What is the most likely diagnosis and what is its definition?

C. How can we manage the patient?

D. What is the equipment used to assist ventilation in picture B?

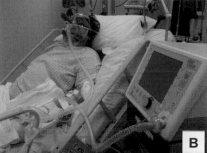

Q1.2
This man had a chronic discharge from his abdominal wall.

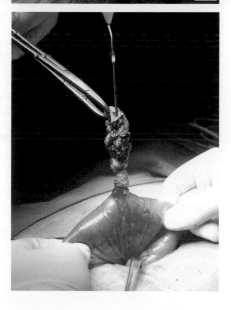

A. What does this intra-operative picture show?

B. What is the definition and natural history of this pathology?

C. What are the possible causes of this pathology?

D. What investigations can be done pre-operatively?

E. What are some reasons that might prevent patients from recovering from this condition?

Answers

A1.1

A. There is an endo-tacheal tube in position, with a central venous catheter inserted via the right internal jugular vein and bilateral fluffy infiltrates in the lungs.

B. Acute respiratory distress syndrome (ARDS) secondary to systemic sepsis.
   1. A known precipitating cause.
   2. Acute onset of symptoms.
   3. Hypoxia refractory to oxygen therapy.
   4. New, bilateral infiltrates in the CXR.
   5. No cardiac failure with fluid overload.

C. Maximal respiratory support with removal of the primary precipitating source of sepsis, which is the liver abscess in this patient.

D. Bilevel mechanical ventilatory support. It allows the patient to breathe spontaneously at two levels of positive end-expiratory pressure (PEEP).

A1.2

A. Isolation and excision of an enterocutaneous fistula tract. Methylene blue dye and a metallic probe are used to isolate the fistula tract so that the entire tract may be excised.

B. A fistula is an abnormal communication between two epithelial-lined surfaces or viscus. In the absence of distal obstruction, most fistulas will close spontaneously.

C. Trauma/injury to the bowel, Crohn's Disease, abscess, diverticulitis or an inadvertent suture left in the bowel wall after surgery.

D. Computed Tomographic (CT) scans can be used to rule out an abscess collection or any inflammatory process within the fistula opening. A fistulogram may identify multiple or branched-tracts.

E. High-output effluent, infection, presence of foreign material, malignancy and poor nutrition.

Q1.3
The 72-year-old lady has had abdominal surgery in the past.

A. What can be seen in these pictures?

B. What factors may predispose one to develop the condition?

C. What may be contained in this lump?

D. What are the indications for emergent surgery?

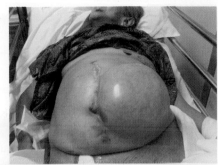

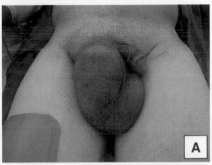

Q1.4
This patient presented with persistent right groin discomfort.

A. What is the condition shown in picture A?

B. What would you perform to obtain more information about the patient's condition?

C. What information would it provide?

D. What is shown in picture B?

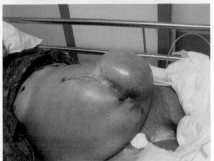

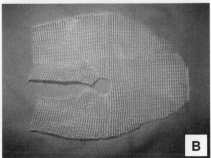

Answers

A1.3

A. Incisional hernia.

B. Poor wound healing.

(**patient factors**) malnutrition, old age, malignancy, immunosuppression, steroids, infection, radiotherapy and obesity.

(**surgeon factors**) poor surgical technique and suture breakage.

C. Any visceral organs (most commonly small or large bowel and omentum).

D. Pain, irreducibility, intestinal obstruction and peritonism which may suggest ischemia of the contents in the sac.

A1.4

A. Right inguinal scrotal lump.

B. Attempt to "get above the lump/mass" or feel the spermatic cord.

C. In adults, if you can get above the cord or feel it, then it is a scrotal or testicular mass. If not, it is an inguinal hernia until proven otherwise.

D. A prosthetic mesh. There are many types of meshes available for the repair of hernias, with various shapes, sizes and materials.

After reduction of the viable contents and hernia sac, the weak posterior wall is reinforced with a tension-free deployment of the mesh. The mesh allows for the scar-plate formation of the posterior wall, thus providing support to prevent the recurrence of a direct hernia.

Q1.5
A procedure had been performed for these patients.

A. What has been inserted into these patients?

B. What are the indications for such use?

C. What two complications can be seen in pictures A and B?

D. What are the other complications which may arise from such a procedure?

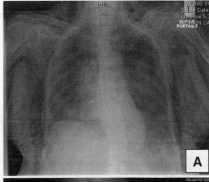

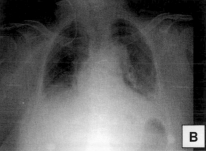

Q1.6
A 40-year-old male presented with sudden onset of severe epigastric pain.

A. What does this chest X-ray show?

B. What is your diagnosis?

C. What do you expect to find on clinical examination?

D. What other radiological signs may be present?

E. What are the possible causes of this condition?

F. Outline your management.

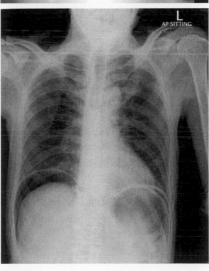

Answers

A1.5

A. Central venous catheters.

B. 1. Administration of intravenous fluids or blood products.
   2. Monitoring intravascular volume and central venous pressure.
   3. Parenteral nutrition.
   4. Blood sampling.

C. 1. Subcutaneous emphysema.
   2. Mal-position – the tip of catheter is in the right subclavian vein instead of the superior vena cava.

D. Haemorrhage, pneumothorax, thrombo-embolic phenomenon and infection.

A1.6

A. The sitting/erect film shows free gas under the diaphragm.

B. Perforated viscus.

C. Tenderness and guarding of the distended abdomen.

D. A visible falciform ligament, Rigler's sign (both sides of the bowel are seen due to the free gas) or free air in triangular shapes between loops of bowel.

E. It is due to a perforated hollow viscus. Perforated peptic ulcer disease (most common), colon cancer or diverticular disease.

F. This patient will have systemic sepsis. He will be dehydrated due to poor oral intake and the loss of fluid into the 3rd space. Resuscitation includes fluid resuscitation, intravenous antibiotics, urinary catheterisation and emergent surgery.

Q1.7
This patient had emergency surgery after presenting with abdominal distension and vomiting.

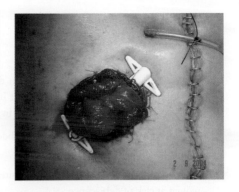

A. What procedure had been performed on this patient?

B. How do you think this patient first presented?

C. How was the abdomen closed?

D. What complications may develop at the stoma?

Q1.8
A 50-year-old man underwent emergency surgery for epigastric pain of acute onset.

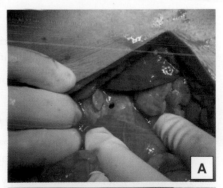

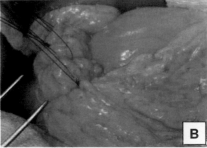

A. What pathology can be seen in picture A and what surgery is being performed in picture B?

B. What physical signs would the patient have presented with?

C. How can we confirm the need for emergency surgery?

D. What further procedures need to be carried out during the surgery?

E. What post-operative management should be considered?

Answers

A1.7

A. A loop colostomy has been created to de-function or divert the large bowel (loop colostomies use a key/bridge to hold it in position on the abdominal wall, unlike an end colostomy). They can also be used in elective surgery.

B. Colonic obstruction. Apart from the abdominal distension, he would be constipated and have a tender abdomen.

C. Primary closure with deep-tension sutures, which are used to buttress an abdominal wound at risk of dehiscence.

D. Early: necrosis and bleeding.
   Late: retraction, parastomal hernia, prolapse or stenosis.

A1.8

A. Picture A shows an upper midline incision with the liver at the superior aspect. A perforated duodenal ulcer is seen. Picture B shows a Graham omental patch repair.

B. Peritonitis leading to generalised abdominal tenderness and abdominal wall board-like rigidity.

C. Presence of free gas in the abdomen on an erect chest X-ray.

D. Peritoneal lavage of the subphrenic spaces, paracolic gutters and pelvis. Inadequate lavage would give rise to intra-abdominal abscesses.

E. *Helicobacter pylori* eradication therapy and follow-up gastroscopy to ensure healing of the ulcer.

Q1.9
This is an erect chest X-ray of a 70-year-old man.

A. What can be seen in the X-ray in picture A?

B. What sign is this?

C. What other condition can mimic the appearance of a pneumoperitoneum?

D. What can be seen in the mediastinum?

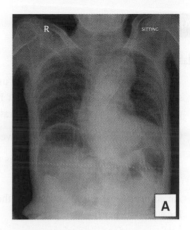

Q1.10
This is a 60-year-old man who underwent emergency surgery.

A. What can be seen in picture A?

B. What are the possible causes?

C. How will the patient present?

D. How can we manage the patient?

E. What can be seen in picture B?

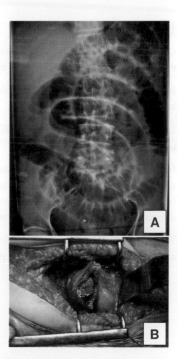

Answers

A1.9

A. The appearance of intra-colonic air under the right diaphragm. This is often due to a shrunken liver. Gas under the right hemidiaphragm is often mistaken as free intra-peritoneal gas suggestive of a perforated viscus.

B. Chilaiditi's sign (transverse colon over the liver simulating free gas).

C. Subphrenic abscess, basal atelectasis that mimics the contours of the hemidiaphragm and cysts in pneumomatosis coli.

D. An aortic stent in place (as seen by the radio-opaque wire mesh). This was performed for a thoracic aortic aneurysm.

A1.10

A. Dilated small bowel. This is evident from the valvulae conniventes in the jejunum and "featureless" characteristics of the ileum. No colonic dilatation is seen.

B. Adhesions, inguinal hernias, femoral hernias, caecal tumour, small bowel tumour, and bezoars.

C. Intestinal obstruction (abdominal colic and distension, vomiting and absolute constipation).

D. Initial management includes nasogastric tube decompression; and fluid and electrolyte resuscitation. Surgery is needed if there are obvious reversible causes (e.g. hernias) or the obstruction does not resolve. In some cases, intestinal obstruction due to adhesions may resolve with conservative management.

E. The patient had operative intervention for intestinal obstruction, which was caused by a phytobezoar. An enterotomy was performed and the phytobezoar removed.

Q1.11
This 65-year-old lady had a painful lump in her right groin.

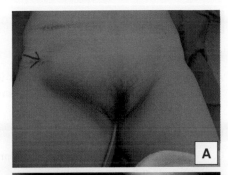

A. What are the differential diagnoses of a groin lump, seen in picture A?

B. Bowel sounds are heard over the lump; and it disappears when the patient is supine. What is this condition?

C. What is the incidence of femoral hernias?

D. What are the boundaries of the femoral canal?

E. Why are they often irreducible?

F. What are the surgical approaches for a femoral hernia repair?

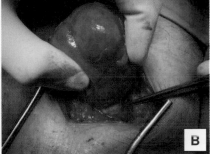

Q1.12
A 75-year-old man with atrial fibrillation presented with an acute onset of abdominal pain.

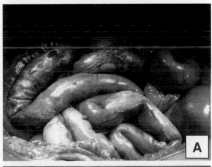

A. What can be seen in picture A?

B. What are the causes of the condition?

C. What is the classical symptomatology?

D. What is the investigation of choice?

E. What procedure had been performed in picture B?

F. What is the prognosis?

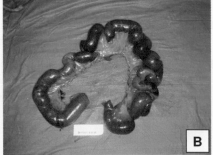

Answers

A1.11

A. Inguinal and femoral hernias, enlarged inguinal lymph nodes, sapheno varix, and femoral artery aneurysm. In males, cysts of the cord and un-descended testes have to be considered.

B. A reducible right groin hernia.

C. Femoral hernias are uncommon and represent 2–4% of all groin hernias (inguinal hernias are still more common).

D. Cooper's ligament posteriorly, inguinal ligament anteriorly, femoral vein laterally and lacunar ligament medially.

E. Compared to inguinal hernias, the neck of a femoral hernia is narrow and the surrounding tissues are not easily stretched (as seen in picture B).

F. Inguinal, pre-peritoneal and femoral approaches.

A1.12

A. Laparotomy showing evidence of ischaemic bowel.

B. Emboli from the heart, acute mesenteric arterial or venous thrombosis, and low-flow states of the mesenteric vessels.

C. "Pain – out of proportion to physical examination." (sentence ambiguous-check author)

D. If the patient is in stable condition, a mesenteric angiogram may be helpful. If there is a high index of suspicion, urgent laparotomy without prior investigation is usually necessary.

E. Resection of the segment of ischaemic bowel. A re-look laparotomy within 24 or 48 hours may be necessary to evaluate the viability of the remaining bowel.

F. The mortality is high, often due to the delay in establishing the diagnosis and the patient's co-morbid problems. Intestinal decompensation can follow extensive resection of the small intestine due to the reduction of the absorptive area and greatly reduced transit time.

Q1.13
This equipment can be found in the surgical ward.

A. What is this?

B. What is it used for?

C. How is it deployed?

D. Name the potential complication associated with the larger balloon.

E. What precautionary measure can one take to avoid this complication?

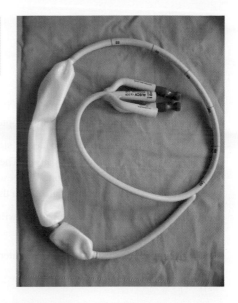

Q1.14
The patient is a 46-year-old man with a history of hepatitis C, who presented with haematemesis.

A. What is being performed?

B. What is the pathogenesis?

C. What is the most common cause of the condition?

D. What factors are predictive of bleeding in this context?

E. How can the bleeding be stopped?

F. How can we prevent recurrent bleeds?

G. What other options can be considered if endoscopic treatments fail?

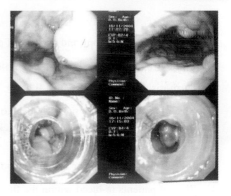

Answers

A1.13

A. A Sengstaken-Blakemore tube.

B. It is an oro- or nasogastric tube used in the management of upper gastrointestinal haemorrhage due to bleeding from oesophageal varices.

C. The gastric balloon is inflated in the stomach with 150 mls of dilute contrast for radiological confirmation of position. The inflated balloon is gently pulled up against the gastro-oesophageal junction. The oesophageal balloon is then inflated. Markings on the tubing indicate the distance from the distal end of the oesophageal balloon.

D. Prolonged deployment of the balloon will lead to pressure necrosis or the rupture of the oesophagus.

E. Releasing the oesophageal balloon at intervals.

A1.14

A. Emergency gastroscopy and banding of esophageal varices (blue rubber bands).

B. Portal hypertension leading to porto-systemic shunting.

C. Cirrhosis (alcohol and hepatitis B or C).

D. Size of varices (directly proportionate to the vessel wall tension), red wheal markings on the varices (from decreased wall thickness), severity of liver disease and persistent alcohol abuse.

E. Injection sclerotherapy or balloon tamponade using a Sengstaken Blakemore tube.

F. 70% of patients re-bleed within the first year. Beta-blockers reduce this risk by half. With variceal treatment, the incidence is reduced by a further half.

G. Transjugular Intrahepatic Portosystemic Shunting (TIPS), surgical shunt (partial/selective) or oesophageal transection.

Q1.15
The patient in picture A was diagnosed with cancer and had an umbilical lump.

The patient in picture B presented with vomiting and an acutely painful lump over the umbilicus.

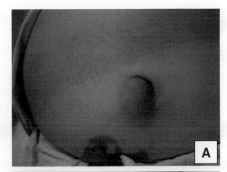

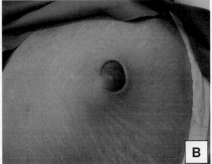

A. What is the diagnosis of the condition in picture A?

B. What is its significance?

C. What can be seen in picture B?

D. What is the treatment for the patient in picture B?

Q1.16
This 29-year-old obese diabetic man presented in a state of septic shock, requiring resuscitation in the Intensive Care Unit.

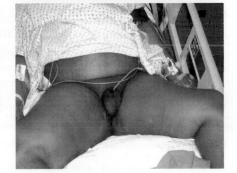

A. What is the diagnosis?

B. What are the usual causative organisms?

C. Which group of patients is susceptible to this condition?

D. How should this condition be treated?

Answers

A1.15

A. The Sister Mary Joseph sign, refers to a palpable nodule bulging into the umbilicus as a result of metastasis from a cancer in the pelvis or abdomen. This patient had ovarian carcinoma with metastatic spread to the umbilical lymph nodes.

B. Gastrointestinal malignancies (most commonly gastric cancer, colonic cancer or pancreatic cancer) account for about half of underlying sources. Gynaecological cancers account for about one in 4 cases (primarily ovarian cancer and also uterine cancer). Proposed mechanisms for the spread of cancer cells to the umbilicus include direct transperitoneal spread, via the lymphatics which run alongside the obliterated umbilical vein, hematogenous spread, or via remnant structures such as the falciform ligament, median umbilical ligament, or a remnant of the vitelline duct.

C. An irreducible and strangulated para-umbilical hernia.

D. Emergency exploration, resection of the necrotic visceral organs and repair of the hernia.

A1.16

A. Necrotising infection of the perineum (Fournier's gangrene) usually caused by a mixed infection of both aerobic and anaerobic bacteria. They present with systemic toxicity and pain over the perineum. Cellulits is seen in the patient but they may present with crepitance and extensive necrosis under relative normal skin.

B. Synergistic flora of the anorectal and urogenital area (streptococcus, clostridia, and non-hemolytic streptococcus).

C. Immuno-compromised patients (e.g. diabetics, alcoholics and malnourished patients).

D. They are associated with high morbidity and mortality. Aggressive surgical debridement and broad spectrum antibiotics is necessary.

Q1.17
A 45-year-old man developed sudden onset of interscapular back pain, associated with some chest pain. He was sweaty and short of breath.

A. Describe the abnormal findings in the picture A.

B. What can be seen in picture B and what is the diagnosis?

C. How is it classified?

D. What is the aetiology?

E. What complications can develop?

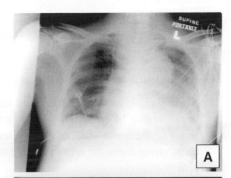

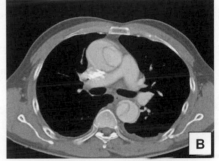

Q1.18
A 20-year-old man suddenly experienced right-sided pleuritic pain.

A. What is the diagnosis?

B. What is its pathogenesis?

C. Who are most at risk of developing this condition?

D. What physical findings are associated with this condition?

E. How do we manage this patient?

F. The patient suddenly becomes breathless and cyanosed. How should he be managed?

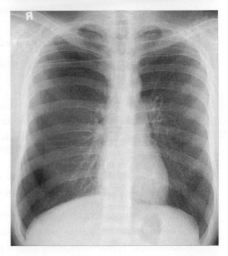

Answers

A1.17

A. Widened mediastinum and opacification of the left lung.

B. Acute aortic dissection. Weakness of the aortic wall resulting in an intimal medial tear, allowing blood to track under pressure through and/or out with the various layers of the aortic wall. A re-entry tear may form resulting in a "double-barrel" aorta, giving rise to the appearance of a tennis ball on the CT scan.

C. DeBakey classification:

Type 1 – affects both ascending and descending.
Type 2 – affects ascending only.
Type 3 – affects distal to the left subclavian artery.

D. Hypertension (most important), Marfan's syndrome, bicuspid aortic valve and cystic medial necrosis.

E. Cardiac tamponade, aortic insufficiency, aortic branch occlusion, leading to ischaemia (e.g. stroke, paraplegia, renal, bowel or lower limb insufficiency).

A1.18

A. Right primary spontaneous pneumothorax.

B. A rupture of an apical pleural bleb. Blebs are considered to be congenital defects in the alveolar wall.

C. Two groups of patients are most at risk. The first consist of fit young adults, often tall, thin young men in whom congenital apical blebs are bilateral. The second group of patients belong to those suffering from emphysema with air trapping and bulla formation.

D. Tachypnoea, tracheal deviation to the contra-lateral side, decreased breath sounds hyper-resonance of right chest and diminished movement of the chest wall.

E. Initial management would involve a thoracostomy (chest drain). These pneumothoraces are often recurrent unless specific surgical treatment is undertaken in the form thoracoscopic apical bullectomy and/or pleurodesis with talc or tetracycline.

F. Suspect a tension pneumothorax. Immediate decompression with a large-bore hypodermic needle is mandated.

Q1.19

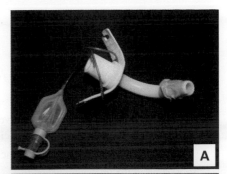

A. What can be seen in picture A?

B. When should it be used?

C. What can be seen in picture B and what kind of clinical scenario could have led to it?

D. What are the other possible complications which may arise as a result of using the apparatus?

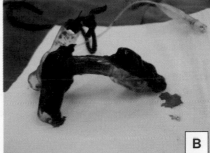

Q1.20
The contents of this bag were administered intravenously to a patient recovering from gastrointestinal surgery.

A. What is contained in this bag?

B. What are the daily nutritional requirements for adults?

C. When should it be used?

D. What are the possible complications which may arise as a result of its use?

E. What is re-feeding syndrome?

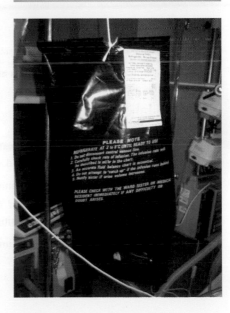

Answers

A1.19

A. A tracheostomy tube with a cuff.

B. Elective or emergency settings.

Ventilatory insufficiency – prolonged ventilation and pulmonary diseases. They help to reduce anatomical dead space and facilitate tracheobronchial lavage.

Airway obstruction – trauma (maxillofacial) and infection (epiglottitis).

Protection of the tracheobronchial tree – after oropharyngeal surgery or head injury.

C. Post-tracheostomy bleeding leading to clot formation around and in the lumen of the tube. This led to airway compromise and required a removal and change of tracheostomy tube.

D. Immediate: haemorrhage, loss of airway, local structure damage (carotid, recurrent laryngeal nerve, esophagus, brachiocephalic vein), apnoea and misplacement.

Late: tracheitis, tracheal necrosis, stenosis, obstruction, displacement and fistula formation.

A1.20

A. Total parenteral nutrition (TPN).

B. The two main components are calories and protein, the former as glucose or fat and the latter as amino acids.

Proteins: 1–1.5 g/kg/day

Calories: 25–30 kcal/kg/day

C. Severe malnutrition, inability to swallow, high output fistula, sepsis, severe pancreatitis, Short Bowel Syndrome and severe Crohn's Disease.

D. (catheter-related): Line sepsis and pneumothorax.

(nutrition-related): Fatty infiltration of the liver, electrolyte/glucose abnormalities, loss of gut barrier, acalculous cholecystitis and re-feeding syndrome.

E. Decreased serum potassium, magnesium and phosphate after re-feeding a starving patient.

Q1.21
The patient is a 52-year-old man who is on immunosuppresion therapy.

A. What does the patient in picture A have in his forearm and what is it used for?

B. What are the potential complications?

C. What surgery did he have over the lower abdomen, based on picture B?

D. What are the possible complications following this surgery?

E. How might transplant rejection present?

F. What kind of immunosuppressive therapy does the patient require?

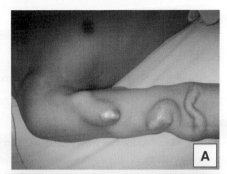

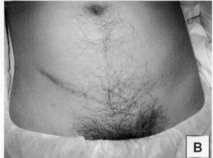

Q1.22
The patient is a 36-year-old lady who presented with abdominal distension.

A. What are the possible causes of abdominal distension?

B. How is ascites confirmed clinically?

C. What are the causes of ascitis?

D. What further investigation should be performed?

E. What information can be obtained from the investigation?

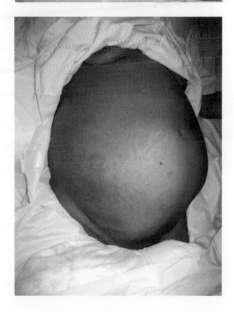

Answers

A1.21

A. Arteriovenous fistula for access for haemodialysis.

B. Thrombosis, aneurysm and high-output cardiac failure.

C. Renal transplantation.
    The donor kidney is transplanted into an extraperitoneal site in the pelvis. The donor renal artery is anastomosed to the recipient's internal or external iliac artery, the donor renal vein to the external iliac vein and ureter into patient's bladder.

D. (Surgical) – thrombosis, urine leak, lymphocele and anastamotic stenosis.
    (Rejection) – hyperacute, accelerated acute, acute and chronic.

E. Tenderness over the graft, reduced urine output and rising serum creatinine.

F. Corticosteroids, azathiaprine and cyclosporine.

A1.22

A. Fluid, fat, flatus, foetus and solid mass.

B. Flank dullness, shifting dullness and a fluid thrill.

C. Common: chronic liver disease, right heart failure, intra-abdominal malignancy and hypoalbuminnaemia.
    Less common: nephrotic syndrome, tuberculosis and chylous ascitis.
    This patient has ascitis secondary to tuberculosis.

D. A peritoneal tap. It may be diagnostic or therapeutic.

E. **Cytology**: presence of malignant cells.
    Protein: transudate or exudate.
    Microbiology: exclude bacterial infection.

Q1.23
The patient underwent surgery on his small intestine and this lesion was found.

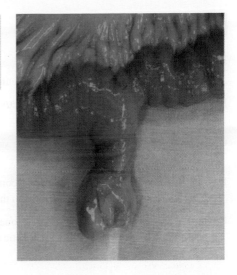

A. What can be seen in this intra-operative picture?

B. What is its origin?

C. Where is it usually located?

D. What are the rules of 2s?

E. How do they present?

Q1.24
This 60-year-old man underwent pelvic surgery 6 days ago. He complained of a painful right calf.

A. What is the cause of his leg pain?

B. What other clinical signs may support the diagnosis?

C. How can we confirm the diagnosis and what is the mode of management?

D. The patient suddenly complains of respiratory distress. What is the probable diagnosis?

E. What additional tests would you carry out to confirm the turn of events?

F. What can be seen in picture B?

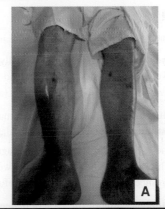

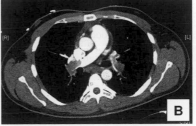

Answers

A1.23

A. Meckel's diverticulum in the terminal ileum.

B. Remnant of the omphalomesenteric duct/vitelline duct, which connects the yolk sac with the primitive midgut in the embryo.

C. About 2 feet from the ileocaecal valve on the anti-mesenteric border of the small bowel.

D. Incidence of 2%, Male 2 times more common, present before the age of 2 years, 2 inches long and its location 2 feet from the ileocaecal valve.

E. Most are asymptomatic but occasionally they may present with intestinal haemorrhage, intestinal obstruction, peptic ulcer disease or diverticulitis.

A1.24

A. Deep vein thrombosis.

B. They are often silent and clinically apparent in 30% of cases. Other signs include swelling, tenderness, erythema and evidence of dilated superficial veins in the right lower limb as compared to the left (as seen in picture A).

C. Ultrasound Doppler and duplex imaging of the calf veins, venography and D-dimer test (breakdown products of coagulation).

   The mainstay treatment is anticoagulation to prevent clot propagation. This can be achieved with low molecular weight heparin or warfarin. Thrombolysis and thrombectomy will not be very useful unless there is impending gangrene.

D. Pulmonary embolism. 20% of patients with DVT will develop a pulmonary embolism and up to 40% may be fatal.

E. ECG, arterial blood gases, ventilation-perfusion lung scan and a spiral CT thorax.

F. Embolism in the right main pulmonary artery.

Q1.25

A. What can be seen in pictures A and B?

B. What are they used for?

C. What is the pathophysiology of a
    thrombosis?

D. What other measures can be used or
    undertaken to prevent thrombosis?

E. What are the complications of
    thrombosis?

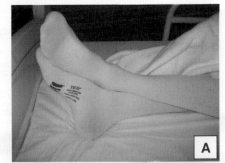

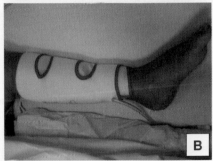

Q1.26
The patient had an
appendectomy a week ago.

A. Describe what you see in the picture.

B. What complication has developed?

C. How can it be classified?

D. What clinical signs and symptoms
    would the patient have?

E. How can the condition be managed?

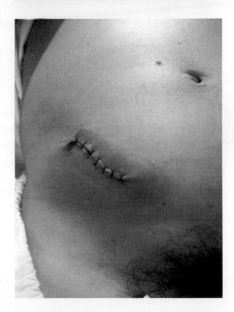

Answers

A1.25

A. Anti-thrombo-embolic stockings (A) and an intermittent pneumatic compression device (B).

B. Peri-operative prophylaxis of lower limb deep vein thrombosis.

C. Virchow's triad. Endothelial damage, hyper-coagulability, venous stasis. Risk stratification can be done, based on operative risk factors, patient risk factors and history of thrombophilia.

D. Early ambulation, anticoagulation (low molecular weight heparin or un-fractionated heparin) and hydration.

E. **Early** – Fatal or non-fatal pulmonary embolism and caerula phlegmasia dolens or albicans.

   Late – Post-phlebitic limb, venous claudication and chronic venous ulceration.

A1.26

A. An incision in the right iliac fossa. The wound has closure with interrupted sutures. There is a surrounding erythema.

B. Surgical site infection (SSI).

C. Superficial – involving skin and subcutaneous tissue.
   Deep – involving soft tissue layers (muscle or fascial).
   Organ specific – involving the anatomical structure operated on.

D. Calor (heat), rubor (redness), tumour (swelling), dolor (pain) and purulent discharge.

E. Antibiotics for treatment of systemic sepsis, lay-opening and irrigation of the wound to drain any collections. It should be allowed to heal by secondary intention.

Q1.27
These equipment were used by a patient who had undergone a total gastrectomy.

A. What can be seen in picture A?

B. How is it useful in the post-operative period?

C. What is the desired measurement?

D. What is seen in picture B and how does it assist the patient in recovery?

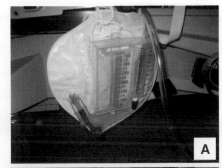

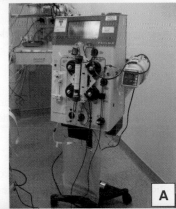

Q1.28
These are modes of renal replacement therapy.

A. When does one need renal replacement therapy? Describe the indications.

B. What equipment is shown in picture A?

C. What equipment is shown in picture B?

D. What is the principle behind the mode in picture B?

E. What are the advantages and disadvantages of each mode?

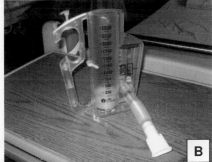

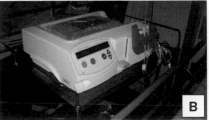

Answers

A1.27

A. Hourly urinary collection to measure the urine output of the patient.

B. Surgery provides a "stress response," which lowers renal perfusion. Open abdominal surgery also increases insensible water loss. The urine output is a reflection of glomerular filtration rate (GFR), which corresponds to renal blood flow and thus the hydration status of the patient.

C. The minimum acceptable urine output is 0.5 ml/kg/hour.

D. An incentive spirometer. It allows the patient to document tidal volume and he will have an "incentive" to increase it.

    Patients often do not have full inspiration due to the pain from abdominal incisions and subsequently develop basal atelectasis of the lungs, which is a common cause of post-operative fever. If not addressed, early atelectasis may progress to pneumonia.

A1.28

A. Uraemia, metabolic acidosis, hyperkalaemia and fluid overload.

B. Haemodialysis (HD).

C. Peritoneal dialysis (PD).

D. The fluid and solute transport characteristics of the peritoneum serve as a dialysis membrane. The fluid instilled in the peritoneal cavity undergoes solute removal and ultra-filtration is achieved.

E. In PD, there is better maintenance of constant serum levels of urea, creatinine and electrolytes, better blood pressure control and the dialysate can provide nutrition. The patient is independent and can take care of his own renal replacement which can be done at home.

    In HD, a shorter time for the procedure is required but it is normally facilitated in a specialised centre.

Q1.29
The 20-year-old boy presented with chest discomfort.

A. What can be seen in the scans?

B. How is the mediastinum divided anatomically?

C. How else might the condition present?

D. What are the differential diagnoses?

E. How do we manage the condition?

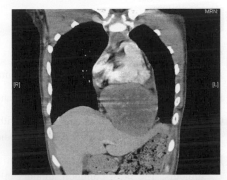

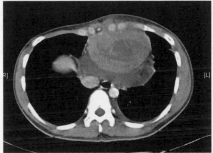

Q1.30
This is the CT film of a 50-year-old chronic smoker who presented with cough and hemoptysis.

A. What is the most likely diagnosis?

B. What are the two main histological types?

C. What diagnostic test can you perform to obtain histological diagnosis prior to surgery?

D. List three treatment modalities.

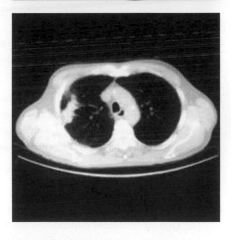

Answers

A1.29

A. A large tumour in the anterior mediastinum.

B. It is divided into four regions: superior, anterior, middle and posterior.

C. If they are large, they may present with compression of the superior vena cava, oesophagus and trachea, requiring immediate attention.

D. Primary lymphomas, teratomas, germ cell tumors, thymomas and neurogenic tumours. The most common tumours in the mediastinum are secondary metastatic deposits in the mediastinal lymph nodes (usually from lung, oesophagus, stomach and breast). This patient had a poorly differentiated neurogenic tumour.

E. Obtain a histological diagnosis. Treatment will be tailored according to the type of tumour.

A1.30

A. Lung cancer. It is the leading cause of cancer in men and the second most common cancer in women. There is an increased risk of lung cancer of up to 15 to 25 times for smokers.

B. Small cell lung cancer (SCLC) and non-small cell lung cancer (NSCLC). This distinction is important because the treatment varies; non-small cell lung carcinoma (NSCLC) is sometimes treated with surgery, while small cell lung carcinoma (SCLC) usually responds better to chemotherapy and radiation.

C. Computer tomography guided fine needle aspiration cytology, bronchoscopy or thoracoscopy.

D. Surgery, radiation and chemotherapy are the three main methods of cancer treatment. The type of treatment depends on the size, extent of the disease, the type of lung cancer and the general health of the patient.

Q1.31

A. What are the advantages and disadvantages of laparoscopic surgery (picture A)?

B. What are contraindications of this mode of surgery?

C. What gas is used to create a pneumoperitoneum and what complications may develop?

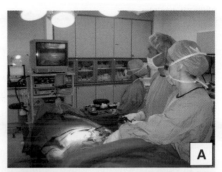

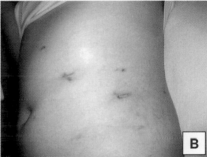

Q1.32

This patient underwent 3 abdominal operations within a week after being involved in a traffic accident.

A. How was the abdominal wall in picture A closed?

B. Why was the abdominal wall closed in this manner?

C. What can be seen in picture B?

D. In what other situations would this method of closure be considered?

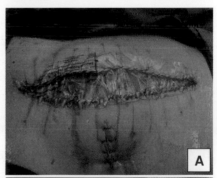

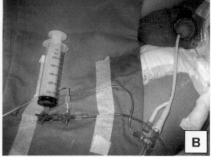

Answers

A1.31

A. Laparoscopic surgery is associated with smaller wounds (picture B), less post-operative pain and quicker wound healing leading to early mobilisation of the patient.

Disadvantages include the need for special equipment and extra training, the need for good hand-eye coordination and loss of tactile feedback during surgery.

B. Patients with sub-optimal cardiac and respiratory status may not tolerate the pneumoperitoneum, which splints the diaphragm and decreases venous return. Patients who have had previous abdominal surgeries are likely to have intra-abdominal adhesions as well as those who are pregnant; in both cases, working space in the abdomen is reduced.

C. Carbon dioxide is used. Oxygen is not used as it is flammable. Rarely does carbon dioxide embolism develop.

A1.32

A. Laparostomy closure with a Bogota bag.

B. To prevent abdominal compartment syndrome. Increased abdominal compartment pressure with the compromise of respiratory (splinting of diaphragm), cardiovascular (decreased pre-load and increased after-load) and renal perfusion.

C. The abdominal pressure is measured indirectly from intra-vesical pressures through a urinary catheter and a pressure transducer.

D. To facilitate repeated laparotomies (e.g. debridement of a necrotic pancreas or re-look for trauma).

Chapter 2

TRAUMA

Q2.1
This man was hit by a bus. He complained of pain over the right chest.

A. Describe the chest X-ray findings in picture A.

B. What is this diagnosis?

C. What is the initial management for this patient?

D. What is the subsequent management for this patient, based on picture B?

E. What are the indications for surgical intervention?

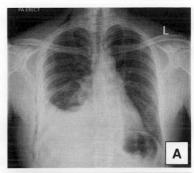

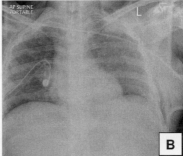

Q2.2
A man fell off his motorcycle. He felt breathless and examination revealed central cyanosis and paradoxical movement of his right chest with crepitus.

A. What abnormalities are seen in the X-ray?

B. What is the likely cause of the clinical findings and how does it affect lung ventilation?

C. What other injuries may occur with this type of chest trauma?

D. How can we manage this injury?

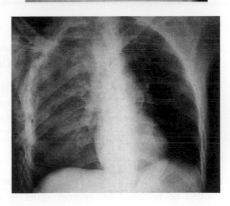

Answers

A2.1

A. There is a fluid level in the right thoracic cavity with right rib fractures (7th to 9th) and subcutaneous emphysema.

B. Right haemothorax.

C. **ABC**: Secure **A**irway; maintain **B**reathing (ventilation) and adequate **C**irculation.

D. Chest tube insertion. It is inserted in the "safe area" of the chest. This is a triangular area, which is the thinnest region on the chest bordered by the posterior border of the pectoralis, mid axillary line and nipple line.

E. Worsening haemothorax. This is evident from the haemodynamic and ventilatory instability of the patient and/or blood drainage from the chest tube (>1.5 litres of blood on initial placement of the thoracostomy or persistent >200 mls/hour of blood for 4 hours).

A2.2

A. Multiple rib fractures with flail segment, radio-hyper-density due to pulmonary contusion and subcutaneous emphysema in the right chest.

B. The paradoxical movement of the chest is highly suggestive of a right flail chest (two separate fractures in three or more consecutive ribs). In spontaneously breathing patients, the portion of the thoracic cage that has lost bony continuity retracts inward during inspiration.

C. Pneumothorax and haemothorax.

D. Adequate ventilation, humidified oxygen and adequate analgesia. Unstable fractures can be managed by internal splinting (internal pneumatic stabilisation) or open reduction and internal fixation with prosthesis.

Q2.3
A man sustained acceleration-deceleration blunt chest trauma following a motorbike accident. The blood pressure readings in both arms were different.

A. What is the abnormality seen in the CXR and what does it suggest?

B. What is the most common initial presentation?

C. What are the possible clinical signs?

D. How can we confirm the diagnosis?

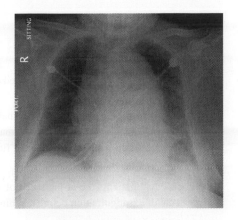

Q2.4
A man was involved in a traffic accident. He had neck pain and was unable to move his lower limbs.

A. What do we look out for when examining the patient?

B. What precautions should be taken?

C. What abnormalities are seen in the X-ray?

D. What other clinical findings could you expect in the patient?

E. What is seen in picture B?

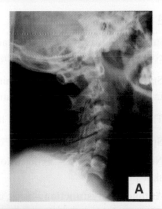

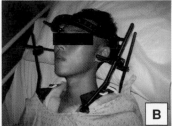

Answers

A2.3

A. A widened mediastinum with right-sided displacement of the trachea. It is suggestive of blunt injury to the thoracic aorta.

Up to 15% of patients may have a normal chest X-ray. Abnormal signs include a left pleural effusion, depression of the left main bronchus, right ward displacement of the oesophagus (with a nasogastric tube), first rib fractures, apical cap and loss of the aorto-pulmonary window.

B. Shock. Most patients die at the scene of injury. 80% of patients with a torn thoracic aorta die of exsanguination before reaching the hospital.

C. They may have upper extremity hypertension, unequal upper extremity pressures, loss of lower extremity pulses and an expanding haematoma at the root of the neck.

D. A high index of suspicion is needed. It can be confirmed by a CT scan if the patient is stable.

A2.4

A. Inspect the neck for external trauma and palpate the spine for step-off. Perform a complete neurological examination of all the extremities.

B. Suspect a spinal injury and minimise additional spinal injury. This can be done by in-line cervical spine immobilisation with a cervical collar and spinal board.

C. There is a fracture dislocation of the cervical spine at the C6–C7 level.

D. **Spinal shock** – Flaccidity, areflexia, loss of anal sphincter tone and priapism.

Neurogenic shock – hypotension, paradoxical bradycardia and flushed dry warm skin.

Autonomic dysfunction – ileus, urinary retention and poikilothermia.

E. This halo external fixation of an unstable cervical spine fracture.

Q2.5
This patient was stabbed in the abdomen. His blood pressure was 90/60 mmHg and was tachycardic.

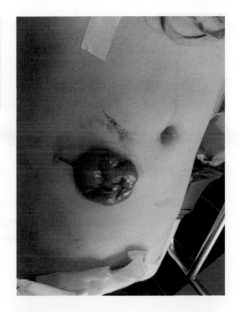

A. What is seen in the picture?

B. How should this patient be managed?

C. Is there a role for diagnostic peritoneal lavage (DPL)?

D. Is there a role for focused abdominal sonography for trauma (FAST)?

E. What is the definitive procedure for the patient?

Q2.6
A 30-year-old motorcyclist was involved in a traffic accident. He had gross haematuria and was in haemodynamic shock.

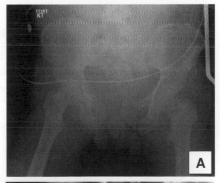

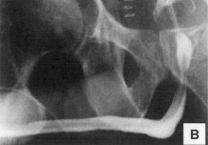

A. What is seen in picture A?

B. What could have caused the shock?

C. What investigation may be done to confirm and treat the condition?

D. Is there a role for mechanical stabilisation?

E. Can a urinary catheter be inserted?

F. Which radiological investigation was performed in picture B and what can be seen?

Answers

A2.5

A. Evisceration of the small bowel.

B. Resuscitate the patient based on Advanced Trauma Life Support (ATLS) principles –
    ABC (airway, breathing and circulation) and AMPLE (**A**llergies, **M**edication, **P**ast
    medical history), **L**ast meal and **E**vents-description of the injury.

C. No.

D. No.

E. Exploratory laparotomy. With this type of injury, we have to assume that there is
    other visceral organ damage and a careful and thorough examination of the intra-
    abdominal organs would be needed. The eviscerated part of the bowels needs to be
    returned to the abdominal cavity.

A2.6

A. Unstable open book fracture of the pelvis with separation of the left sacroiliac joint.

B. Trauma patients with displaced pelvic fractures have high incidence of other
    associated injuries. Pelvic fractures can cause shock by bleeding from exposed
    cancellous bone surfaces, pelvic veins and pelvic arteries.

C. Selective catheter angiography can be done to identify and embolise the source of
    bleeding if it was from a major vessel.

D. Open-book and vertical shear fractures with displacement may benefit from pelvic
    stabilisation (external wrap or fixation). This decreases bleeding by decreasing the
    pelvic volume, providing a tamponade effect and opposing the fractures, thus
    promoting clot formation.

E. Yes, unless it suggests urethral injury and blood is observed at the penile meatus.

F. Ascending urethrogram. An intact urethra.

Q2.7
This man suffered fractures on the 9th, 10th and 11th rib on his left ribcage.

A. What is seen in picture A?

B. How might this patient have presented?

C. When is emergency surgery indicated?

D. What is seen in picture B?

E. What are the complications associated with the removal of the organ?

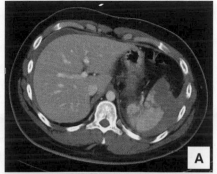

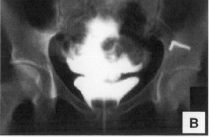

Q2.8
This man was resuscitated after being involved in a traffic accident. A urinary catheter was inserted.

A. What can be seen in picture A?

B. Which organ/s are likely to have been injured?

C. When would you be wary of inserting a urinary catheter?

D. Which radiological investigation was performed in picture B and what abnormality can be seen?

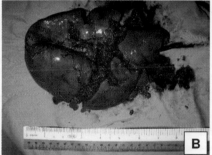

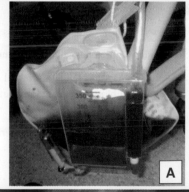

Answers

A2.7

A. Based on this history, we have to strongly consider the possibility of a splenic injury. When the patient is haemodynamically stable, a CT scan may be used to evaluate intra-abdominal visceral injuries. The CT scan shows a splenic laceration with blood around it. Contrast leak into the abdomen suggests-on-going bleeding.

B. Hypovolaemic shock due to a haemoperitoneum, peritonitis from extravasated blood and Kehr's sign (referred shoulder tip pain resulting from left diaphragmatic irritation).

C. When there is haemodynamic instability; evidence of persisting bleeding or other intra-abdominal injuries, surgical intervention is necessary.

D. A shattered spleen (the most common solid organ damaged in blunt abdominal trauma).

E. Overwhelming post-splenectomy infection (OPSI). Patients with splenectomy are advised to take lifelong oral antibiotic prophylaxis.

Post-splenectomy patients may also develop thrombocytosis.

A2.8

A. Urometer catheter bag showing gross haematuria.

B. The kidneys, ureters, bladder or urethra are likely to have been injured.

C. When there is a suspicion of urethral disruption – retention of urine, massive perineal swelling and blood in the urethral meatus.

D. Ascending urethrogram/cystogram. There is extravasation of contrast into the peritoneal cavity, suggesting intraperitoneal bladder rupture.

Q2.9
A 27-year-old female pillion rider was involved in a road traffic accident.

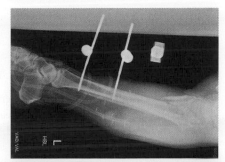

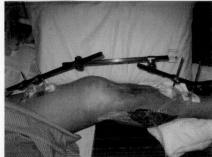

A. Describe the injury sustained.

B. What has been performed for the patient?

C. What complications are associated with this condition and its treatment?

Q2.10
A patient was admitted to hospital with a Glasgow Coma Score of 5 following a road traffic accident.

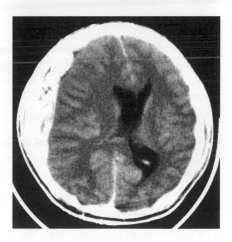

A. What is the initial management of a brain-injured patient?

B. What does the CT scan show?

C. What is the management if the patient is hypotensive?

D. What is the significance if this patient develops anisocoria (unequal pupils)?

E. What is the surgical management?

Answers

A2.9

A. Comminuted fracture of her upper tibia. There is an associated soft tissue swelling.

B. External fixation of the fracture. External fixation is usually used when internal fixation is contraindicated – often to treat open fractures, or as a temporary solution. A fasciotomy has also been performed, evident from the suction dressing over the medial aspect of the calf.

C. Osteomyelitis, delayed union or non-union tibia, pin track infection/loosening, ankle stiffness and Compartment Syndrome.

A2.10

A. Initial management and resuscitation using ATLS principles as in any trauma situation. After that, neurological examination is needed. It includes checking for level of consciousness, eye pupil and motor examination. Also, look out for cervical spine injury.

B. Acute Subdural Haemorrhage (SDH).

C. Hypotension in patients with head injury frequently accompanies other injuries. We need to rule out other sources of bleeding before assuming that the condition is simply due to brain injury.

D. It is a surgical emergency. There is stretching of the ipsilateral third nerve indicative of raised intracranial pressure.

E. Craniotomy and evacuation of the clot.

Chapter **3**

HEPATOBILIARY

Q3.1
The patient is a 43-year-old man who had jaundice for 2 weeks.

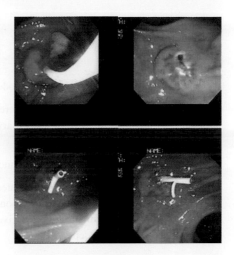

A. Which part of the upper gastrointestinal tract is revealed in this endoscopic procedure?

B. Which diagnostic and therapeutic procedures have been performed?

C. How would this patient present?

D. What are the potential complications of performing this procedure?

Q3.2
This is a elderly lady with a long history of alcohol consumption.

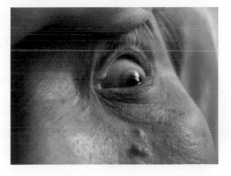

A. What clinical sign does she have?

B. How do we classify this condition?

C. Which blood investigations can be done to confirm the diagnosis?

D. What complications may this patient encounter during surgery?

E. How can we prevent these complications?

Answers

A3.1

A. The papilla in the second part of the duodenum.

B. Endoscopic retrograde cholangio-pancreatogram (ERCP), sphincterotomy of the papilla to facilitate removal of any biliary duct stones and the placement of stent to ensure drainage of the bile.

C. Jaundice, and signs and symptoms of pancreatitis or cholangitis.

D. Sphincterotomy of the papilla is associated with bleeding and perforation (commonly retroperitoneal). Pancreatic duct irritation during cannulation of the biliary tree can lead to pancreatitis. Patients are often given prophylactic antibiotics as the procedure may be associated with sepsis.

A3.2

A. Jaundice as seen through the yellowing of the sclera. Bilirubin levels of above 50 umol/l are usually clinically detected.

B. **Pre-hepatic**: caused by haemolytic anaemia.
    Hepatic: caused by hepatitis.
    Post-hepatic: obstructive/surgical jaundice caused by biliary obstruction.

C. In obstructive jaundice, there will be elevated serum conjugated bilirubin, increased alkaline phosphatase and gamma-glutamyltransferase, and increased conjugated bilirubin in the urine.

D. Coagulopathy (failure to absorb vitamin K from the gut affects the synthesis of clotting factors ii, vii, ix and x), renal failure (hepato-renal syndrome), poor wound healing and increased susceptibility to infection.

E. Administer intra-muscular vitamin K, adequate peri-operative hydration, additional peri-operative nutrition and appropriate coverage with broad-spectrum antibiotics.

Q3.3
This 56-year-old Chinese man presented with progressive jaundice.

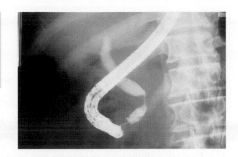

A. What investigative procedure is this and what does it reveal?

B. What is the most likely diagnosis?

C. Who are most commonly affected by this condition?

D. What are the risk factors?

E. How can this pathology be classified?

F. How can we manage this patient?

Q3.4
This abdominal CT scan was performed for a 53-year-old lady who had severe abdominal pain.

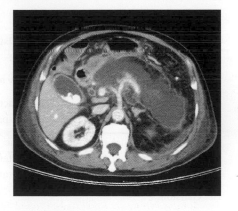

A. What 2 abnormalities are revealed in this scan?

B. What is your diagnosis?

C. What is the pathophysiology?

D. What are her symptoms?

E. What is the most likely aetiological factor of this patient?

F. What kind of blood investigation can confirm the diagnosis?

G. What is the prognosis of the patient's condition?

Answers

A3.3

A. The ERCP study shows a filling defect with shouldering in the middle portion of the common bile duct.

B. Cholangiocarcinoma. The history of jaundice; being progressive, suggests a malignant stricture. The lesion is in the middle of the bile duct.

C. There is a slight male preponderance with a peak incidence in the sixth decade.

D. They are common in the Far East where parasitic infections are endemic. It is associated with *Opisthorchis viverrini* infestation. Weak associations include bacterial-induced endogenous carcinogens derived from bile salts and ductal calculi.

E. They are best classified according to their anatomical site of origin: intra-hepatic, proximal (right and left) and its confluence (Klatskin) and distal (distal CBD and peri-ampullary).

F. Curative surgery provides the best prognosis. Post-operative adjuvant radiotherapy has been reported to provide survival benefit. Cholangicarcinomas are generally unresponsive to chemotherapy.

A3.4

A. The contrast-enhanced CT shows gallstones and a pancreatic collection with no enhancement of normal pancreas.

B. Extensive pancreatic necrosis secondary to acute pancreatitis.

C. The inflammation and oedema of the acute pancreatitis progressed with subsequent devitalisation of the pancreatic and peri-pancreatic tissue.

D. Severe abdominal pain radiating to the back. Abdominal examination may reveal diffuse abdominal tenderness with distension, and guarding and hypoactive bowel sounds. She may be febrile, tachycardic and dehydrated.

E. Gallstones.

F. Serum amylase and lipase. Up to 30% of patients with pancreatitis have normal amylase levels ("burned-out" pancreas).

G. 80% of patients with mild pancreatitis recover. Mortality is due to early multiple organ failure or sepsis from infected pancreatic necrosis.

Q3.5
This 46-year-old man had an episode of pancreatitis 3 months ago.

A. What can be seen in picture A?

B. What can be seen in picture B?

C. What is shown in the gastroscopy in picture C?

D. What is the diagnosis?

E. What kind of symptoms do you think the patient has?

F. What procedure is performed in picture D?

G. In what other way can this condition be managed?

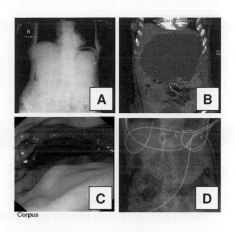

Q3.6
The patient is a 24-year-old man who had suffered a blunt injury to his abdomen.

A. What can be seen in picture A?

B. Is this a common occurrence?

C. What investigation was performed in picture B and what does it indicate?

D. What is the abnormality seen in picture B?

E. What serum blood test may useful in the diagnosis of this condition?

F. What surgical options are available?

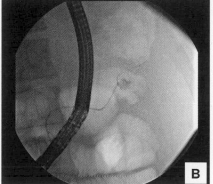

Answers

A3.5

A. Lack of bowel shadows and a generalised radio-dense appearance in the upper abdomen.

B. The coronal CT of the abdomen shows a large homogenous mass in the abdomen.

C. The inability to distend the abdomen despite insufflation of air due to extrinsic compression by the mass.

D. A pancreatic pseudocyst is a circumscribed collection of fluid rich in blood, and necrotic tissue, typically located in the lesser sac of the abdomen. They occur 6 weeks after an episode of acute pancreatitis.

E. Abdominal mass, early satiety, gastric outlet obstruction, abdominal discomfort and sepsis from secondary infection of the cyst.

F. Endoscopic internal drainage into the stomach with 2 double pig-tail tubes. The cyst had decompressed significantly.

G. Open or laparoscopic external or internal surgical drainage.

A3.6

A. Injury to the pancreas. There is a full thickness laceration in the body of the pancreas.

B. They are uncommon due to the position of the pancreas in the retroperitoneal area. It occurs in 2% of blunt and 10% of penetrating visceral injuries. During abdominal trauma, the pancreas is compressed against the vertebral column.

C. When there is a suspicion of a disruption of the pancreatic duct, an ERCP was performed to check its integrity.

D. Leakage/extravasation of contrast indicate a disruption of the pancreatic duct.

E. Up to 50% of patients who have sustained pancreatic injuries have an elevated serum amylase level.

F. Ligation of the proximal pancreatic duct elements and preserve pancreatic tissue or a distal pancreatectomy.

Q3.7
A 50-year-old man presented
with vague abdominal pain
and weight loss.

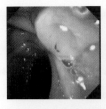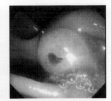

A. What can be seen, based on the
   endoscopy procedure?

B. What can be seen on the
   pancreatogram?

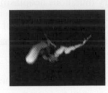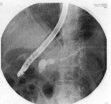

C. What is the diagnosis?

D. What can be done at ERCP to further
   investigate this condition?

E. What is the management of this
   condition?

Q3.8
The patient presented with
right-sided abdominal pain
and fever.

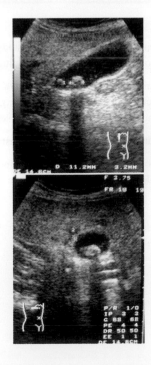

A. What investigation was performed and
   what does it show?

B. Why is this mode of investigation the
   most sensitive way of detecting this
   pathology?

C. How should the patient prepare
   himself for this investigation?

D. What other findings should we look
   for during the investigation?

Answers

A3.7

A. A patulous papilla that resembles a "fish eye" with mucus extruding from the orifice.

B. A segmentally dilated pancreatic duct without stricturing.

C. Intraductal papillary mucinous neoplasm (IPMN) of the pancreas.

D. We can obtain cytology by aspiration of the duct contents or brushings. The cytology examination may reveal mucin and floating epithelial cells with varying degrees of atypia.

E. With a high index of suspicion that the neoplasm has malignant potential, curative surgical resection should be aimed for.

A3.8

A. Trans-abdominal ultrasound study of the hepato-biliary system.
    Stones in the gallbladder. An ultrasound detects 90% of gallstones.

B. Gallstones are highly reflective and cast a distal acoustic shadow (as seen in the picture). The small and mobile gallstones may not be detected in CT or MRI scans. They have to be calcified to be seen in X-rays.

C. The patient has to fast for at least 6 hours so that the gallbladder is distended.

D. Stones in the common bile duct (CBD), diameter of the CBD, thickness of the gallbladder and peri-cholecystic fluid.

Q3.9
The patient is a 40-year-old lady who had a cholecystectomy.

A. What can be seen in picture A?

B. How could the patient have presented?

C. What can be seen in picture B?

D. Which two approaches to cholecystectomies are available?

E. What are the indications for an intra-operative cholangiogram?

F. What are the complications associated with this surgery?

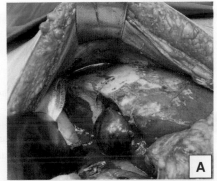

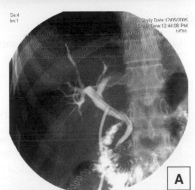

Q3.10
This lady had surgery for gallstone disease.

A. What surgery was performed on this patient?

B. What is the purpose of the tube drain?

C. How long should the tube be kept there?

D. What procedure was performed prior to the removal of the tube in picture A?

E. What if some gallstones are retained?

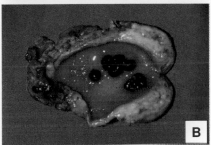

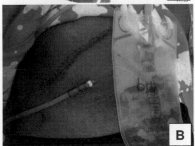

Answers

A3.9

A. A gangrenous gallbladder.

B. Biliary colic, cholecystitis, cholangitis and pancreatitis.

C. Gallbladder with gallstones.

D. Laparoscopic or open method. The laparoscopic method is the most common method of cholecystectomy as it is safe and has all the advantages of a minimally invasive procedure.

E. Any suggestion of the concurrent presence of a ductal stone (jaundice, hyperbilirubinaemia, elevated alkaline phosphatase, choledocholithiasis on ultrasound) and defining the biliary ductal anatomy.

F. Leakage of bile from the cystic duct or gallbladder bed, injury to the common bile duct leading to a biliary stricture and jaundice due to retained stones in the biliary tree.

A3.10

A. Cholecystectomy, common bile duct exploration and closure of the duct over a T-tube. Picture A shows the T-tube being deployed in the common bile duct and picture B shows the surgical wound with the tube being externalised through the skin and draining bile in the bag.

B. When there is concern that a primary closure of common bile duct could lead to a stricture formation, a T-tube is used.

C. 14 to 21 days. It allows for a tract between the biliary duct and skin to develop and for the oedema secondary to surgical biliary duct manipulation to resolve.

D. A check cholangiogram through the T-tube to ensure no biliary obstruction and good flow of contrast from the proximal biliary tree into the duodenum. After removal of the tube, the tract biliary-cutaneous tract should close naturally.

E. With a T-tube in place, they can be extracted with a Dormia basket down the tube (Burhenne manoeuvre).

Q3.11
The patient is a 69-year-old lady who presented with loss of weight and obstructive jaundice.

A. What can be seen in picture A?

B. What else might she complain of?

C. What are the possible causes?

D. What procedure was performed on her (picture B) and what was its indication?

E. What alternative procedure can be performed?

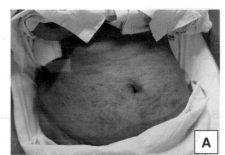

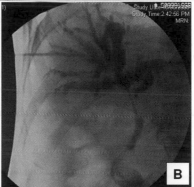

Q3.12
The patient is a 40-year-old man who is a chronic alcoholic.

A. What is the lesion seen in the oesophagus through endoscopy in picture A?

B. What can be seen in picture B?

C. What is their pathogenesis and what are the causes?

D. What other complications might develop?

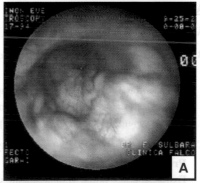

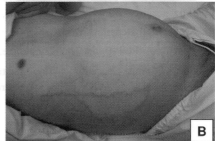

Answers

A3.15

A. Multiple hypodense lesions in both lobes of the liver.

B. Hepatic abscesses.

C. Bile duct infection from ascending cholangitis, ascending pylephlebitis from any inflammatory process within the abdomen, haematogenous spread from bacteriaemia, direct extension from intra-abdominal suppuration and cryptogenic.

D. Pyogenic and amoebic.

E. The position of the liver beneath the costal margin masks abdominal tenderness. These lesions often present as pyrexia of unknown origin.

F. Initial management is usually non-surgical with administration of intravenous antibiotics. Closed percutaneous drainage under radiological guidance can be performed. Multiple abscesses usually respond better to open surgical drainage.

A3.16

A. Hepatocellular carcinoma (HCC).

B. Hepatic adenoma.

C. Based on the segments described by the French anatomist Couinaud, there are 8 segments, each considered a functional unit with its own hepatic artery, portal vein, bile duct and hepatic vein. This lesion is in segment 5 and 6.

D. It is contra-indicated as it may cause seeding of malignant cells to the skin surface during percutaneous biopsies, thus "upstaging" the disease. Furthermore, bleeding can be a potential complication during the procedure as it is a vascular tumour.

E. First, exclude metastatic disease. Second, ensure that there is adequate functional reserve liver tissue (these patients often have chronic liver disease). Excision of the cancer can be performed with a 1–2 cm margin of unaffected liver tissue.

Q3.17

This is a specimen taken from a 50-year-old Chinese man who is a hepatitis carrier. He underwent a hemi-hepatectomy.

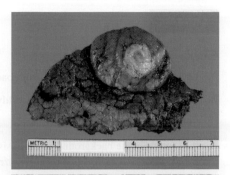

A. What is the most likely diagnosis?

B. How common is this condition?

C. Which geographic areas have the highest incidence?

D. What are the likely aetiological factors in Asia?

E. What macroscopic types are there?

F. What can be seen in the histological specimen?

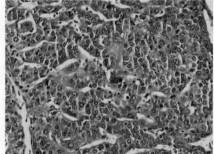

Q3.18

The 33-year-old lady presented with fever, jaundice and pain in the right hypochondrium.

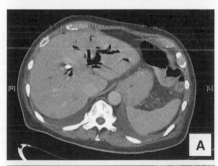

A. What can be seen in picture A?

B. How are her symptoms best described? What is the diagnosis?

C. Which group of organisms is involved?

D. What is the prognosis of this condition?

E. How should we manage this patient?

F. What procedure was performed in picture B?

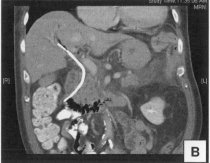

Answers

A3.17

A. Hepatocellular carcinoma (HCC) with background cirrhosis.

B. It is the most common malignancy worldwide.

C. Sub-Saharan Africa and Far East Asia.

D. It develops in the background of cirrhosis (cirrhomimetic), in particular, the Hepatitis B or C virus, but can originate in non-cirrhotic hepatic parenchyma.

E. Unifocal (large mass replacing part of the liver), multifocal (tumour nodules involving different parts of the liver) and diffuse infiltrative (tumours permeate and diffusely enlarge the liver).

F. Thickened trabeculae of neoplastic hepatocytes separated by sinusoids.

A3.18

A. The intrahepatic biliary ducts are dilated.

B. The classic Charcot's triad. Acute bacterial cholangitis. Confusion and hypotension can occur in patients with suppurative cholangitis, producing Reynold's pentad.

C. Gram negative organisms (*Escherichia Coli*, *Klebsiella*, *Pseudomonas*, *Enterobacter* and *Proteus*).

D. Mortality can occur in up to 10% of patients with severe cholangitis.

E. Prompt treatment involving rehydration, intravenous antibiotics and ductal drainage.

F. The biliary tree was decompressed with an internal biliary stent.

Q3.19
This 35-year-old Chinese man underwent surgery after recurrent episodes of cholangitis.

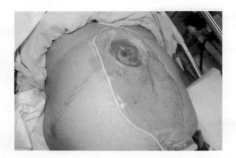

A. What is seen in this patient?

B. What are the contents of the bag?

C. What surgery has been performed?

D. What is the probable diagnosis?

E. Why is the surgery necessary?

F. What is the prognosis for the patient?

Q3.20
This is a 36-year-old alcoholic who presented with vague abdominal pain radiating to the back.

A. What can be seen in picture A?

B. What can be seen in picture B?

C. How do we confirm the diagnosis?

D. How do we manage the condition?

E. What scoring systems can be used to assess the condition's severity and prognosis?

F. What are the potential complications?

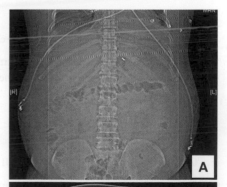

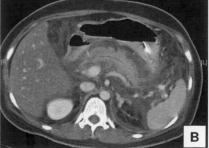

Answers

A3.19

A. A right roof-top incision and a stoma bag situated in the epigastrium.

B. Bile (yellow stain).

C. Hepaticocutaneous jejunostomy.

D. Oriental cholangiohepatitis (OCH). It is a disease characterised by recurrent intra-hepatic pigment stone formation, resulting in biliary obstruction with recurrent cholangitis, dilatation and stricturing of the biliary tree.

E. To facilitate the clearance of stones and infected bile with a choledochoscope at multiple sessions. It can also allow the dilation of intra-hepatic strictures and fragmentation of stones.

F. The most common causes of death in these patients are sepsis, liver failure and complications from cirrhosis.

A3.20

A. Colon cut-off sign. A dilated transverse colon overlying an inflamed pancreas.

B. The CT scan shows acute pancreatitis with peripancreatic inflammation. The pancreas is still well-vascularised and the pancreatic duct is visualised.

C. Elevated serum amylase (>1000 u/ml).

D. Volume resuscitation, analgesia, close monitoring and identify cause to prevent recurrence.

E. Glasgow-Imrie, Ranson and APACHE II.

F. Early: necrotising pancreatitis which can lead to infected necrosis.
Late: pseudocyst.

Chapter 4

COLORECTAL

Q4.1
A 25-year-old gentleman complained of constipation and severe anal pain following defaecation.

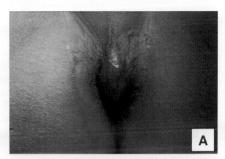

A. What are common causes of perianal pain?

B. What are possible diagnoses, based on picture A?

C. What is the treatment?

D. What procedure was performed in picture B?

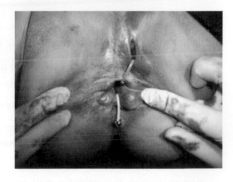

Q4.2
This is a 47-year-old man who complained of perianal pain and discharge.

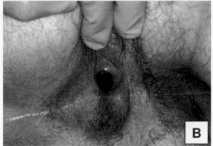

A. What is the diagnosis?

B. Define the condition.

C. What underlying diseases is the condition associated with?

D. How can we classify this disease?

E. How can we manage them?

F. What procedures have been carried out for this patient?

Answers

A4.1

A. Anal fissure, anal fistula, perianal abscess and thrombosed haemorrhoids.

B. Perianal haematoma/thrombosed pile or a perianal abscess. The cause of a perianal haematoma is obscure, but what happens is thrombosis in a subcutaneous vein below the transitional zone. Perianal abscess result from infection of the anal glands in the crypts at the dentate line.

C. It may resolve with symptomatic management, although during this time, they may rupture and ulcerate. If the pain is severe, the haematoma or abscess may be drained.

D. Deroofing of the haematoma with extrusion of the blood clot which is often described as "blackcurrant."

A4.2

A. Anal fistula. There is an external opening at the 1 o'clock position.

B. An abnormal track lined by granulation tissue between the anal canal or rectum and the perianal skin. It can persists following drainage of a perianal abscess.

C. Crohn's Disease, ulcerative colitis or tuberculosis.

D. According to the position of the internal opening in relation to the external anal sphincter (i.e. low-level for an opening below and high-level for an opening above).

E. Low ones can be laid open (fistulotomy). High ones which pass above the anorectal ring or through the sphincter must not be laid open completely as incontinence is likely to result.

F. Seton placement. Insertion of the seton will establish the site of internal opening on re-examination. It also acts as a wick to allow the acute reaction around the track to subside.

Q4.3
A 44-year-old woman complained of bright red rectal bleeding and painful defaecation for 1 month.

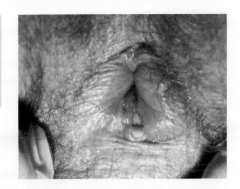

A. What is the diagnosis?

B. What are the differential diagnoses?

C. How can we manage this condition conservatively?

D. Which surgical procedure is appropriate if conservative treatment fails?

Q4.4
A 35-year-old bus driver presented with pain and discharge in the lower back region.

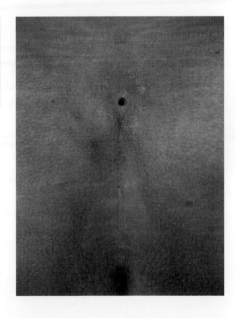

A. What is evident in this patient?

B. What is its aetiology?

C. Who are commonly at risk?

D. How do we treat this condition?

Answers

A4.3

A. Anal fissure – longitudinal tear in the mucosa of the anal canal (90% posterior and 10% anterior). 90% is caused by local trauma from passing hard stools and spasm of the internal anal sphincter.

B. Crohn's Disease, tuberculosis, anal cancer, fistula, cytomegalovirus, herpes simplex virus, chlamydia and syphilis.

C. 90% of cases heal with conservative treatment. Patients are advised to avoid straining when defaecating, increase fibre in their diet, and use stool softeners and local anaesthetic agents. Doctors may also prescribe the use of agents which may promote relaxation of the internal anal sphincter. These include topical nifedipine ointment, topical nitrates calcium channel blockers and Botulinum toxin injection.

D. Lateral internal anal sphincterotomy. This is the partial division of the external sphincter through a small laterally placed stab incision.

A4.4

A. Pilonodal sinus and evidence of previous surgery. These are blind-ending tracks containing hairs in the skin of the natal cleft.

B. It is still not completely understood but it is thought to be an acquired condition. Buttock movement promoting hair migration into a sinus. It may present as an abscess or discharging sinus.

C. Men in the second and third decades of life. It is also more common in those whose occupation involves prolonged sitting.

D. If uncomplicated, advice on good personal hygiene may be adequate. When infected, it is drained with healing by secondary intention. When quiescent, the sinus can be excised. Recurrence rate may be as high as 50%.

Q4.5
These equipments may be used in the outpatient surgical clinic.

A. What is on display in the picture?

B. What is it used for?

C. What is the pathology and how do we classify it?

D. What is an alternative mode of treatment other than the one shown in the picture?

E. How can we prevent a recurrence of the condition?

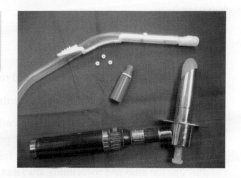

Q4.6
These patients presented with perianal discomfort.

A. What is the diagnosis?

B. What is the symptomatology?

C. What are the predisposing factors?

D. How would you manage this condition?

E. What complications may arise after surgery?

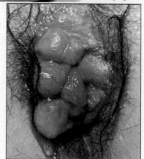

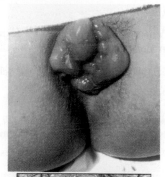

Answers

A4.5

A. Proctoscope, rubber band applicator and rubber bands.

B. Diagnosing and ligating/banding haemorrhoids.

C. Haemorrhoids are engorged vascular cushions found within the submucosa of the anal canal. They are found at constant positions within the anal canal (3, 7 and 11 o'clock). Classification can be made in four degrees, based on whether they prolapse through the anus and reducibility after that.

D. Injection sclerotherapy.

E. Appropriate advice to prevent straining and constipation.

A4.6

A. Prolapsed haemorrhoids (3rd-degree piles are reducible and 4th-degree piles are irreducible).

B. Excruciating pain, bleeding and itch.

C. Prolonged straining at defaecation, constipation and pregnancy.

D. If they are **reducible**, advice on bowel regulation, having a high-fibre diet and avoidance of prolonged straining may be sufficient.

If they are **irreducible**, surgical resection (haemorrhoidectomy) is needed.

E. **Early**: Bleeding, infection and acute retention of urine due to post-operative pain.

Late: Incontinence (injury to the sphincter complex) and anal stricture formation (excess amount of anal mucosa resected, leading to scarring).

Q4.7
This 72-year-old lady complained of a protruding mass at her anus following defaecation.

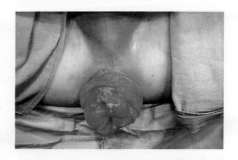

A. What is seen here?

B. What other symptoms might this patient complain of?

C. What is the aetiology of this condition?

D. If conservative treatment fails, what is the surgical management option?

Q4.8
This 45-year-old lady had previous abdominal surgery for intestinal obstruction.

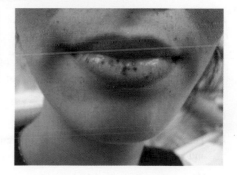

A. What is seen in this patient?

B. What syndrome is this condition associated with?

C. How is it inherited?

D. What is the malignancy potential of this condition/syndrome?

E. What other abdominal complications may occur with this condition?

F. What is the recommended management in view of these possible complications?

Answers

A4.7

A. Rectal prolapse, which is a protrusion from the anus of the rectal mucosa (partial) or rectal wall (full thickness).

B. Pain, bleeding, mucus discharge or incontinence.

C. Rectal intussusception, poor sphincter tone, chronic straining and pelvic floor injury.

D. In a **fit patient**, a transabdominal rectopexy +/− anterior resection may be considered (Wells, Ripstein's and Goldberg-Frykman procedure).

In an **elderly and unfit patient**, a perineal proctectomy can be considered (Delormes, Thiersch or Altheimer).

A4.8

A. Melanin spots on the lips.

B. Peutz-Jeghers Syndrome. This consists of familial intestinal harmatomatous polyps affecting the jejunum and melanosis of the oral mucus membranes and the lips, hands, perianal and umbilical areas.

C. Autosomal dominant.

D. There is an increase risk (10%) of malignancy in the gastrointestinal tract, pancreas and extra-intestinal organs.

E. Haemorrhage into the jejunum or intestinal obstruction due to intussusception.

F. All polyps larger than 2 cm should be removed in view of the risk of malignancy.

Q4.9
This 50-year-old man was investigated for a urinary infection.

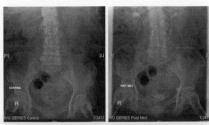

A. What abnormality is seen in these radiological investigations?

B. What is the condition?

C. What are the possible causes of this anomaly?

D. How may the patient present?

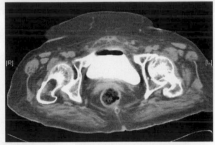

Q4.10
This investigation was done in a 60-year-old man for lower abdominal pain.

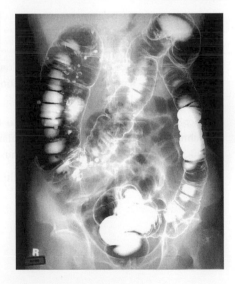

A. What is this radiological examination?

B. Which pathological condition is depicted?

C. What is the pathogenesis?

D. How may this patient present at the emergency department?

Answers

A4.9

A. Air in the bladder.

B. Colovesical fistula.

C. Cancer (bladder or colon) or any inflammatory condition (inflammatory bowel disease, tuberculosis, post-radiation therapy or diverticulitis).

D. Recurrent urine infection, pneumaturia, dysuria or faecal-uria.

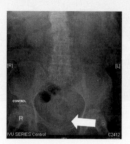 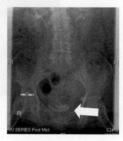

(arrow shows the air in the bladder in both the contrast and non-contrast films)

A4.10

A. Double contrast barium enema.

B. Diverticular disease (Diverticulosis). Common in patients aged 50 years and above with a male: female ratio of 1:1.5. Aetiology is due to a low-fibre diet, leading to increased intraluminal colonic pressure.

C. Increased intraluminal pressure leads to false diverticula in which the mucosa and submucosa protrude through the muscularis propria. It occurs at the anti-mesenteric side where the arterioles penetrate the muscularis.

D. Haematochezia or peritonitis (diverticulitis, diverticular abscess or perforation).

Q4.11
This is a gross specimen of a resected colon from a 25-year-old patient.

A. What is the diagnosis?

B. What is its inheritance pattern?

C. Where is the gene located?

D. What are the chances of this patient developing colon cancer?

E. What other tumours are associated with this condition?

F. What operation was performed for this patient?

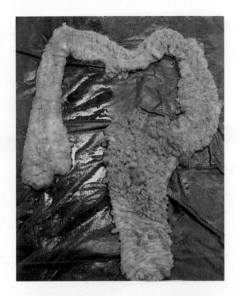

Q4.12
A 68-year-old man was admitted with massive per-rectal bleeding. After resuscitation, the patient underwent urgent colonoscopy.

A. What can be seen from the endoscopy in picture A?

B. What is their distribution in the colon?

C. What is another major cause of massive lower gastrointestinal haemorrhaging?

D. How can we manage this patient?

E. Which surgical procedure was performed in picture B?

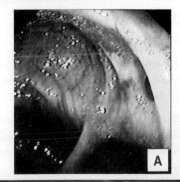

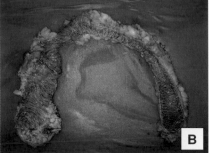

Answers

A4.11

A. Familial adenomatosis polyposis (FAP). It is a general neoplastic disorder of the intestine whereby numerous (>100) polyps are found mainly in the large bowel.

B. Mendelian autosomal dominant. Males and females are equally affected.

C. The Adenomatous Polyposis Coli (APC) tumour suppressor gene is on chromosome 5q21.

D. Carcinoma of the large bowel occurs between 10–20 years after the onset of polyposis. One or more cancers will be found in two-thirds of symptomatic patients.

E. Benign mesodermal tumours (desmoid tumours, osteomas) and epidermoid cysts (Gardners Syndrome).

F. Total colectomy with either end ileostomy, an ileal pouch anal anastomosis (IPAA) or rectal anastomosis.

A4.12

A. Blood and diverticula in the colon. Bleeding diverticular disease.

B. Diverticular disease is found in over 50% of patients over 60 years of age. In the West, there is a predominant left-sided preponderance. In the East, they tend to occur in the caecum and ascending colon.

C. Angiodysplasia. It is a vascular malformation seen in the elderly. They occur in the ascending colon and caecum of elderly patients. They consist of dilated tortuous submucosal veins, and in severe cases, the mucosa is replaced by massive dilated deformed vessels.

D. With conservative management, 80% of diverticular bleeding will stop. If bleeding persists, consider laparotomy and segmental colectomy if the source of bleed is localised. If it is not localised, a total colectomy may be necessary.

E. A total colectomy.

Q4.13
This 25-year-old female who presented with a distended abdomen, non-tender to palpation.

A. What can be seen intra-operatively in picture A?

B. What is the most likely cause?

C. Which procedure was performed in picture B?

D. What additional treatment can be carried out during surgery?

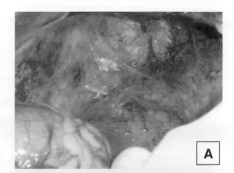

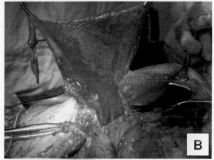

Q4.14
This is a 60-year-old man who was sent to the emergency department.

A. What are the findings in picture A?

B. How would the patient have presented?

C. How would you classify this obstruction (open or closed)?

D. If the obstruction is not relieved, which part of the gut is likely to perforate?

E. What is the most likely cause of the obstruction shown in picture B?

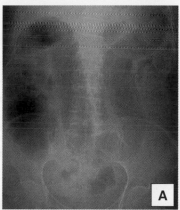

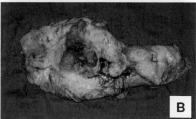

Answers

A4.13

A. Pockets of mucus in the peritoneal cavity (pseudomyxoma peritonei or "jelly belly").

B. Pseudomyxoma peritonei. It is an uncommon tumour known for its production of an abnormal amount of mucus in the abdominal cavity. It is associated with both mucinous and cystic tumours of the ovary and appendix.

A thorough search for a primary tumour. If there isn't one, perform an appendectomy and/or oophorectomy (if there is any suggestion of an ovarian tumour).

C. Radical resection of the parietal peritoneal surface.

D. Intra-peritoneal chemotherapy.

A4.14

A. Dilated ascending and transverse colon.

B. Symptoms of intestinal obstruction. Abdominal distension and constipation.

C. Closed-loop obstruction – A competent ileo-caecal valve allows ingress of luminal content into the loop (n.b. absence of dilated small bowel loops). Thus vomiting (especially faecal contents) may not be a feature.

D. Increase in luminal pressure would be greatest in the caecum, with subsequent impairment of the blood supply, resulting in caecal necrosis and perforation.

E. Carcinoma of the descending colon.

Q4.15
This 46-year-old man underwent a colectomy.

A. What is seen in the gross specimen?

B. How would he have presented?

C. What is the most likely diagnosis?

D. What is seen in the microscopic specimen?

E. What are the principal patterns of the inheritance of colorectal cancer?

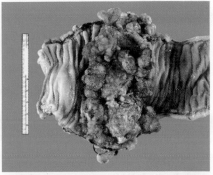

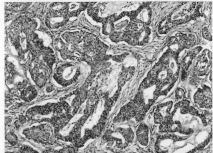

Q4.16
This 45-year-old man had a neoplastic lesion 12 cm from the anal verge on endoscopy.

A. How would he have presented?

B. What is the diagnosis and which staging systems are commonly used for this condition?

C. Where is the proposed development of this lesion?

D. What are the common macroscopic varieties of the original lesion?

E. What are some objectives in the surgical management of a low rectal lesion?

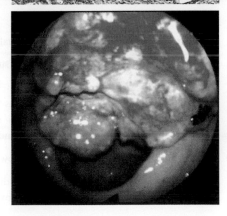

Answers

A4.15

A. A circumferential ulcerated polypoidal lesion.

B. Being circumferential, he probably presented as "napkin-ring" intestinal obstruction.

C. Colorectal cancer.

D. Infiltrating neoplastic glandular structures within fibroblastic stroma.

E. **Sporadic**: most common.

   Inherited: FAP – (accounts for 2%) autosomal dominant.
   HNPCC – (accounts for 5%) autosomal dominant.
   Familial colorectal cancer – runs in families but no gene defect known.
   Syndromes such as Lynch 2 and Li-Fraumeni.

A4.16

A. Per rectal bleeding, tenesmus or intestinal obstruction.

B. Adenocarcinoma of the colon/rectum. Dukes' and TNM (International Union against Cancer).

C. It is likely that all carcinomas start as benign adenomas, the so-called "adenoma carcinoma sequence," where there is an accumulation of about 5–10 stepwise mutations in tumour suppressor genes and oncogenes over a lifetime.

D. Annular, tubular, ulcerative and cauliflower.

E. Radical excision of the rectum (including the mesorectum and associated lymph nodes) with preservation of continence by preserving the anal sphincter.

Q4.17
This 50-year-old man had undergone a radiological investigation.

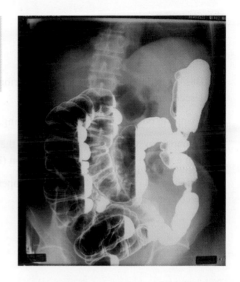

A. What can be seen in this radiological film?

B. How may this patient have presented?

C. How should this condition be managed?

D. If the patient was unfit for surgery, what could be done to relieve the obstruction?

Q4.18
This 44-year-old lady underwent colonoscopy for the investigation of iron deficiency anaemia. The caecum is displayed.

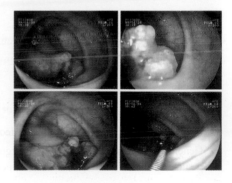

A. Describe the gross pathology seen.

B. What was attempted during the colonoscopy?

C. What is the most probable histology in this area?

D. How would this patient have presented?

E. Which surgical procedure would be recommended?

Answers

A4.17

A. This is a double contrast barium enema showing an "apple core" lesion in the descending colon.

B. Change in bowel habit, per-rectal bleeding, and cramping abdominal pain.

C. Colonoscopy with biopsy can confirm the diagnosis of cancer and stage the disease with a view to curative surgical resection (left hemicolectomy).

D. Endoluminal stenting. If there is impending caecal perforation, an emergency caecostomy may be performed.

A4.18

A. An ulcerating polypoid lesion at the caecum.

B. Tissue biopsy of the lesion.

C. Adenocarcinoma.

D. Abdominal mass, intestinal obstruction or intussusception.

E. Right hemicolectomy with end-to-end ileo-colic anastamosis.

   General principles of oncological surgery include early ligation of the vascular pedicle, no-touch technique, and avoidance of contamination by bowel content.

Q4.19

A 62-year-old man was admitted to hospital for intestinal obstruction and emergency surgery was performed on him.

A. What procedure was carried out, based on picture A and why?

B. What is an alternative procedure?

C. What is the main physiological derangement of small bowel obstruction?

D. What surgical resection was performed on the patient, based on picture B?

E. What is the most probable cause of the obstruction?

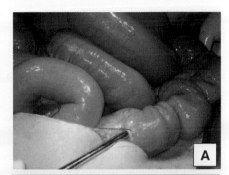

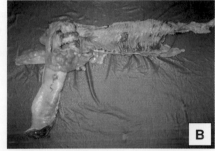

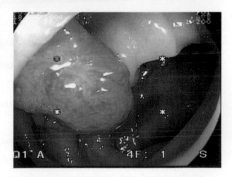

Q4.20

A 45-year-old man underwent sigmoidoscopy for profuse mucus discharge per rectum. A 2 cm lesion was seen in his rectum.

A. What is this lesion?

B. What biochemical abnormality may be associated with this lesion?

C. What is the risk of malignancy?

D. What are the treatment options?

Answers

A4.19

A. On table antegrade decompression on the small bowel. A Savage decompressor had been inserted into the small bowel.

B. Retrograde milking to the contents into the stomach for aspiration via a wide-bore nasogastric tube.

C. There is dehydration and electrolyte loss due to reduced oral intake, intestinal wall oedema leading to defective intestinal nutrient and fluid absorption, losses due to vomiting and sequestration into the small bowel. These patients will need adequate resuscitation and correction of fluid and electrolyte imbalance.

D. Right hemicolectomy. The resection specimen includes the terminal ileum, caecum with appendix and ascending colon.

E. Cancer of the colon.

A4.20

A. Villous adenoma. They are often very large and can occasionally fill the rectum.

B. Hypokalaemia. Villous adenomas secrete mucous high in potassium content which can cause electrolyte and fluid losses.

C. Proportional to the size. Lesions greater than 4 cm have up to 90% chance of malignancy.

D. Small (1–2 cm): endoscopic polypectomy.

Medium (2–4 cm): trans-anal endoscopic microsurgery (TEM), full thickness local excision with suture closure of the defect.

Large (>4 cm): resection of the rectum: either an ultra-low anterior resection or abdomino-perineal resection (APR).

Chapter 5

VASCULAR

Q5.1
A 60-year-old man presented with a vague abdominal mass.

A. What abnormality can be seen in this CT scan?

B. What is the possible symptomatology?

C. How should this patient be managed?

D. What are the potential complications?

E. What surgery has been performed for the patient?

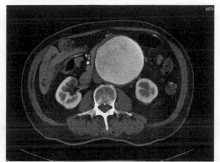

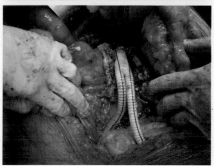

Q5.2
This 70-year-old man had severe back pain.

A. What clinical sign can be seen in picture A?

B. What does the CT scan in picture B reveal?

C. What is the treatment for him?

D. What complications may develop?

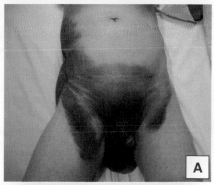

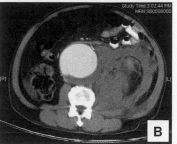

Answers

A5.1

A. Abdominal aortic aneurysm (AAA).

B. 75% of them are asymptomatic. They are often detected during routine radiological examination. Symptomatic AAAs can present due to pressure on adjacent structures, expansion, rupture or distal embolisation.

C. Based on symptoms and size.

   Asymptomatic: if the maximum transverse diameter is <5.5 cm, routine surveillance is recommended.

   If the diameter is >5.5 cm or there is an interval expansion by more than 0.5 cm in 6 months, surgery is advised.

   Symptomatic: urgent surgery is advised.

D. Rupture, trash foot, ureteric or duodenal obstruction (inflammatory AAA) and aorto-duodenal fistula.

E. Open repair of the aneurysm with a bifurcated graft.

A5.2

A. There is bruising over the flanks and suprapubic area. This is Cullens sign-retroperitoneal haematoma associated with a ruptured aneurysm or acute haemorrhagic pancreatitis.

B. It shows a contained retroperitoneal haematoma from a ruptured abdominal aortic aneurysm.

C. This is a surgical emergency. The patient should have large bore intravenous access, blood cross-matched and be consented and prepared for open surgical or endovascular repair.

D. The mortality and morbidity following repair of a ruptured AAA is high. Post-operative complications include cardiac, respiratory and renal failure, abdominal compartment syndrome, mesenteric and limb ischaemia.

Q5.3
This patient presented with bilateral foot pain associated with a recent onset of gangrene of the toes.

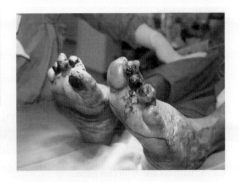

A. What can be seen in the picture?

B. What is it caused by?

C. What is the management?

Q5.4
This man presented with an ache in his lower limb.

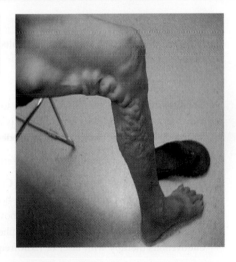

A. What condition does this patient have? Define the condition.

B. Which anatomical distribution area is affected?

C. What is the pathophysiology and what are the predisposing risk factors?

D. What are the potential complications?

E. How should the condition be treated?

Answers

A5.3

A. Bilateral trash feet (acute ischaemia) from microembolism. Note that the gangrene is bilateral.

B. They are due to showers of emboli. The most common source is from the heart (arrhythmias, prosthetic heart valves, valvular heat disease, septic vegetations), abdominal or thoracic aneurysms, aortic atherosclerosis or intra aortic balloon pumps.

C. 1. Correct the source/cause.

2. Management of the gangrene:

Conservative – spirit dressings which allow the lesions to demarcate, anticoagulation if there are no contraindications.

Surgical – If the lesions are infected and wet, transmetatarsal amputation is indicated.

A5.4

A. Varicose veins. They are tortuous dilated prominent superficial veins in the lower limb.

B. Greater saphenous vein.

C. There is venous valve failure leading to backflow in the venous system. Primary varicose veins occur early where there is a strong family history. Secondary varicose veins are due to a post-thrombotic episodes, occupation, parity, age and obesity.

D. Thrombophlebitis, bleeding, venous eczema and venous ulceration.

E. Symptomatic veins should be treated. Conservative measures include avoidance of long periods of standing and support hosiery. Smaller veins may be treated with injection sclerotherapy. Larger veins above the knee usually require high saphenous ligation and stripping of the great saphenous vein. An alternative to stripping is endovenous therapy with laser or radiofrequency ablation.

Q5.5
This diabetic patient presented with pain in the leg of 3 months duration.

A. What condition does the patient have?

B. What is the underlying cause?

C. Describe the features leading to your diagnosis.

D. Which non-invasive test can be performed to determine the extent of reflux?

E. How should this condition be managed?

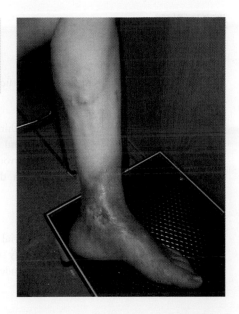

Q5.6
This 49-year-old man complained of discolouration in the legs. He is a chronic smoker.

A. What can be seen in picture A?

B. This patient had his lower limb elevated at 45 degrees. What can be seen in picture B?

C. What is the diagnosis?

D. What other symptoms might he have?

E. What other clinical signs support the diagnosis?

F. Which non-invasive test can be performed to determine the extent of the disease?

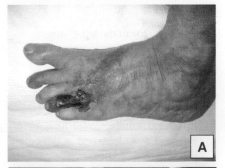

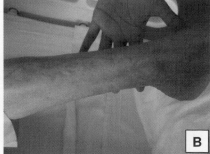

Answers

A5.5

A. Venous ulcer from chronic venous insufficiency.

B. Venous hypertension.

C. The site of the ulcer is in the lower third of the medial aspect of the lower limb ("gaiter area"). The edge is slopping and pale purple in colour. The base is covered by granulation tissue. There are surrounding signs of chronic venous disease (induration, pigmentation, and brown discolouration from lipodermatosclerosis.) There is also evidence of varicose veins.

D. Venous duplex scan.

E. Confirm the diagnosis and exclude arterial and neuropathic causes.
4-layer compression bandaging is mostly successful.
Superficial venous surgery may be considered in some cases.

A5.6

A. Dry gangrene of the left 4th toe.

B. Venous guttering.

C. Chronic limb ischaemia.

D. Intermittent claudication and rest pain (especially at night).

E. Prolonged capillary refill time, absent pulses, arterial ulcers, contractures, positive Buergers test, decreased sensation and proprioception and abnormal ankle-brachial pressure index (ABPI).

F. Arterial duplex scan, CT or magnetic resonance angiography (MRA).

Q5.7

A 50-year-old man presented with sudden onset of pain and numbness in his left foot. He was previously asymptomatic. He has atrial fibrillation.

A. What is the diagnosis?

B. Which vessel is affected in picture A?

C. What other clinical signs may be present?

D. How should the condition be managed?

E. What procedure has been performed in picture B?

F. What complications may develop after the procedure?

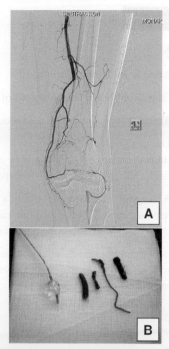

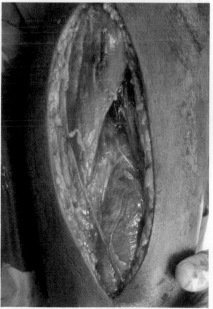

Q5.8

This 30-year-old man had urgent surgery on his lower limb following a road traffic accident.

A. Which procedure has been carried out?

B. What are the indications?

C. What is the pathogenesis of this syndrome?

D. Name the fascial compartments in the calf?

E. What complications may develop?

Answers

A5.7

A. Acute lower limb ischaemia.

B. Embolic or thrombotic occlusion of the popliteal artery.

C. Absent pulses, foot pallor, coldness, paralysis, atrial fibrillation.

D. This is a surgical emergency.
    Heparin anticoagulation should be started.
    Embolectomy, thrombolysis or bypass surgery may be considered.

E. A surgical embolectomy using a Fogarty balloon. Next to the balloon are the removed emboli. This procedure can be performed under local anaesthesia through a groin incision to isolate the common femoral artery.

F. Ischaemic-reperfusion injury. This is systemic process characterised by metabolic acidosis, hyperkalaemia, rhabdomyolysis, cardiac arrhythmias, pulmonary dysfunction and compartment syndrome.

A5.8

A. Fasciotomy of the lower limb.

B. Compartment syndrome from acute ischaemia or following reperfusion.

C. The muscles swell within a tight osseo-fascial compartment. There is an increase in pressure in the compartment greater than the capillary perfusion pressure. The blood supply is interrupted and ischaemia develops. The ischaemia depletes intracellular energy stores and reperfusion leads to oxygen radicals, causing cellular swelling and interstitial fluid accumulation.

D. The four compartments are anterior, lateral (peroneal), deep and superficial posterior compartments.

E. Neurological deficit in the distribution of the peroneal nerve with weak dorsiflexion and numbness in the first dorsal webspace.

Q5.9
These patients sought treatment at the surgical clinic.

A. What is your diagnosis, based on picture A?

B. What is its pathogenesis?

C. What are the possible causes?

D. What can be seen in picture B and what is the management method?

E. What complications may arise from this condition?

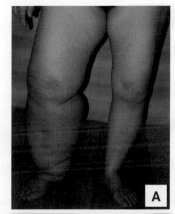
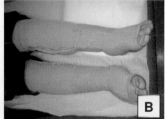

Q5.10
This patient presented with an abnormal gait.

A. What can be observed in this patient and what is your diagnosis?

B. What investigations are appropriate?

C. What are the possible complications?

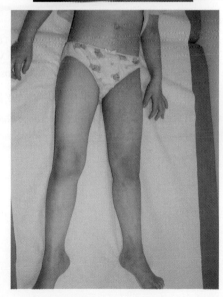

Answers

A5.9

A. Lymphoedema.

B. It is the accumulation of protein-rich fluid in the tissues and is caused by the failure of lymph transport. It is characterised by unilateral limb swelling but can occasionally develop bilaterally.

C. **Primary lymphoedema** – no obvious cause. There are three forms based on age of presentation. *Congenital*; Milroys Disease or praecox (most common), *adolescence* (tarda), and *middle age*.

   Secondary lymphoedema – removal or destruction of the draining lymph nodes by malignancy, infection, surgery or radiotherapy.

D. Compression hosiery. Conservative treatment is the mainstay of treatment. It includes elevation, manual lymphatic drainage, compression hosiery or external pneumatic compression. Surgery is considered in severe cases with complications.

E. Skin ulceration, cellulitis and lymphangitis.

A5.10

A. This patient has discolouration over the left half of her body. Arteriovenous malformation: Parkes Weber or Klippel Trenaunay Syndrome characterised by a port wine stain, varicose veins, bony and soft tissue hypertrophy.

B. MRI, selective angiography, venography and serial skeletal X-rays.

C. Cellulitis, thrombophlebitis, bleeding, ulceration, venous thromboembolism, scoliosis and gait abnormality.

Q5.11
This man suffered a transient ischaemic attack.

A. What kind of lesion can be seen in picture A?

B. What clinical signs may be evident?

C. What symptoms may he experience?

D. What measures may be undertaken to prevent this?

E. What can be seen in picture B?

F. Which cranial nerves may be damaged during this surgery?

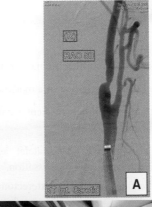

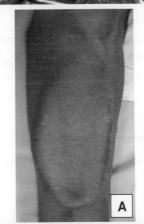

Q5.12
This patient had chronic renal failure.

A. What can be seen in the patient's forearm in picture A?

B. What material is it made of?

C. What complications may develop?

D. What can be seen in picture B?

E. How can we manage the condition?

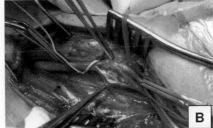

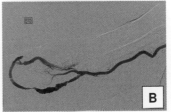

Answers

A5.11

A. A focal stenosis in the internal carotid artery.

B. Carotid bruit suggestive of a moderate to severe stenosis.

C. Contralateral stroke, transient ischaemic attack or ipsilateral amaurosis fugax and retinal artery occlusion.

D. Medical therapy – antiplatelet agents, lipid lowering therapy, antihypertensive medication and smoking cessation.

    Intervention – carotid endarterectomy, carotid angioplasty and stenting.

E. Carotid endarterectomy.

F. Cranial nerves ix, x and xii.

A5.12

A. An antecubital loop arteriovenous graft for haemodialysis.

B. A PTFE (polytetraflouroetylene) graft is anastomosed to the brachial artery and the cephalic or basilic vein in the antecubital fossa.

C. Graft thrombosis, infection, pseudoaneurysm formation, ischaemic steal and high output cardiac failure.

D. Stenosis of the graft.

E. Balloon angioplasty of the stenosis or revision of the graft.

Q5.13
This 20-year-old man with Marfan's Syndrome presented with acute chest pain.

A. What is the diagnosis?

B. What is Marfan's Syndrome?

C. What is the appropriate treatment?

D. What are the risks to the patient if the lesion was left untreated?

E. What other clinical features might the patient have?

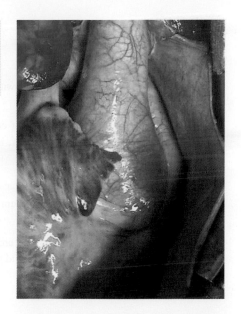

Q5.14
A 25-year-old intravenous drug abuser was bleeding from a tender and expanding mass in his right groin.

A. What is the diagnosis?

B. How may it be confirmed?

C. What complications may arise?

D. How should the condition be treated?

E. What precautions should be taken?

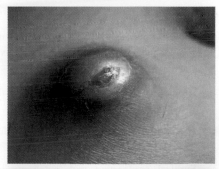

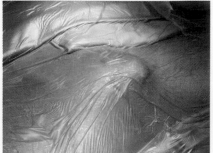

Answers

A5.13

A. Acute Type A aortic dissection as shown by the haematoma seen in the ascending aorta.

B. It is a dominantly inherited disorder of connective tissue where abnormal collagen synthesis affects the basal cement layer, in particular, the musculoskeletal, vascular and ocular systems.

C. Replacement of the ascending aorta.

D. Myocardial infarction, haemopericardium, stroke, rupture, mesenteric and renal or lower limb ischaemia.

E. Blindness due to lens dislocation, high arched palate, aortic valve incompetence and mitral valve prolapse, arachnodactyly and joint weaknesses.

A5.14

A. Femoral pseudoaneurysm. A pseudoaneurysm differs from a true aneurysm in that its wall is made up of organised thrombus only. This patient had punctured his groin vessels repeatedly.

B. Imaging using ultrasound, CT or MRA may confirm the diagnosis and assist in planning for surgery.

C. Bleeding, infection, limb ischaemia, deep venous thrombosis, neuropraxia of the femoral nerve and groin ulceration.

D. Surgical exploration with patch repair or bypass with saphenous vein. If the aneurysm is chronic, triple ligation may be considered. This patient underwent an exploration.

E. The patient should undergo testing for Hepatitis B and C, and HIV.

Q5.15
This 35-year-old man had painful lesions in his hands and feet. He had been smoking 30 cigarettes a day for the past 10 years.

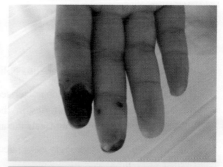

A. What is the diagnosis?

B. Define the condition.

C. What are the aetiological factors?

D. What kind of investigation is appropriate?

E. What is the treatment?

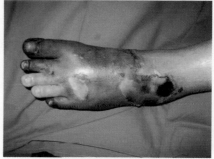

Q5.16
This lady had a deep vein thrombosis.

A. What procedure has been done?

B. What approaches may be used?

C. What are the indications?

D. What complications may develop?

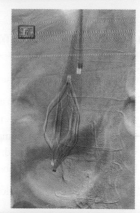

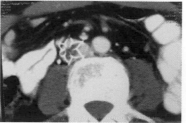

Answers

A5.15

A. Buergers Disease or thromboangiitis obliterans.

B. It is a clinical syndrome characterised by segmental thrombotic occlusions of small and medium sized arteries in the limbs. These are accompanied by dense inflammatory infiltrates that affects the arterial wall.

C. It is unknown but it is strongly associated with smoking.

D. Autoimmune screen, thrombophilia screen, fasting glucose, angiography, echocardiogram.

E. Cessation of tobacco usage, prostacyclin infusion, thrombolysis, amputation and rehabilitation.

A5.16

A. An Inferior Vena Caval (IVC) filter has been placed in the IVC to prevent pulmonary embolus (PE).

B. Trans-jugular or trans-femoral under fluoroscopic guidance.

C. (i) Recurrent DVT/PE despite anticoagulation.

   (ii) Existing contraindication to anticoagulation such as recent gastrointestinal bleeding or stroke; or complication to anticoagulation in patients who have a venous thrombo-embolic disease. Also, as prophylactic use for patients with a high risk of pulmonary embolism.

D. IVC thrombosis with resultant lower limb swelling and IVC filter migration.

Chapter 6

HEAD AND NECK

Q6.1
This patient underwent surgery on the tongue.

A. What is seen in picture A?

B. What is seen in picture B?

C. What are the symptoms of his condition?

D. Which part of the tongue are these lesions more commonly found?

E. What is the etiology?

F. What are the modes of treatment?

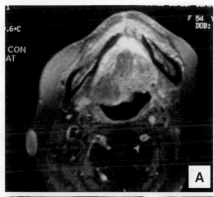

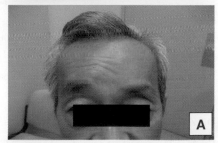

Q6.2
This gentleman had previous head and neck surgery.

A. What clinical sign is evident in picture A?

B. What clinical sign is evident in picture B?

C. What clinical sign is evident in picture C?

D. What are the 2 other branches of the facial nerve?

E. Is this an upper motor neuron lesion?

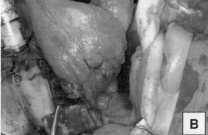

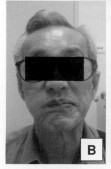

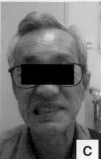

Answers

A6.1

A. The MRI reveals a mass lesion arising from the right aspect of the tongue.

B. Pre-operative tracheostomy for maintenance of airway during surgery and a mandibulotomy to facilitate full exposure, revealing the carcinoma of his tongue.

C. A hard ulcerated mass which bleeds easily. As the tumour grows, it infiltrates the tongue causing increasing pain, and speech and swallowing difficulty.

D. Most (50%) occur in the middle and lateral aspect of the tongue and lower lip. They do not occur commonly on the dorsum.

E. Smoking and alcohol ingestion. Human Papilloma Virus (HPV) is present in up to 15%. Chewing betel nuts and "lime" are important regional cultural influences in India and other parts of Asia.

F. Surgery/radiotherapy or both for small lesions. Localised lesions can be treated surgically. Larger lesions require combination therapy. With treatment, the 5-year survival rate is 50%.

A6.2

A. Weakness of the left frontalis muscle due to palsy of the temporal branch of the facial nerve.

B. Weakness of the left buccinator due to palsy of the buccal branch.

C. Palsy of the mandibular branch.

D. Zygomatic and cervical.

E. No. The temporal branch palsy would be spared in an upper motor neuron lesion (bilateral corticobulbar supply).

Q6.3
This 70-year-old lady presented with a lump under her tongue.

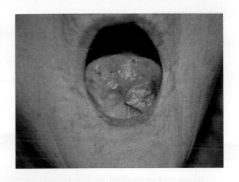

A. Describe the lesion.

B. What tests would you carry out for diagnosis?

C. What are the possible differential diagnoses?

D. What other anatomical region should you examine?

E. What investigation would be useful for further evaluation?

Q6.4
This is a 55-year-old man, a chronic smoker, who had presented with a lump in the neck.

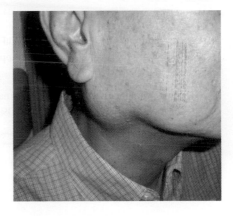

A. Describe the lesion seen on this man?

B. What is the most likely diagnosis?

C. Who does it mostly affect?

D. How should the lump be treated?

Answers

A6.3

A. There is a 3 x 3 cm elevated fungating lesion arising from the dorsal surface of the left side of the tongue.

B. Incisional biopsy under local anaesthesia.

C. Squamous carcinoma or erythroplakia.

D. Full examination of the neck to ascertain any cervical lymph node spread of the disease. Carcinoma of the tongue spreads early to the lymph nodes and up to 15% present with a "lump in the neck."

E. Magnetic resonance imaging (MRI) is better than CT scans for assessing soft tissue spread and the images are not degraded by metallic dental restorations.

A6.4

A. A well-circumscribed, smooth spherical mass arising at the angle of the left jaw. There is no overlying skin change. It appears to arise from the lower pole of the left parotid gland.

B. Warthin's tumour (papillary cystadenoma lymphomatosum) – classically a soft mass arising from the lower pole and up to 30% can be bilateral.

C. Males, 50–70 years. Smokers have a greater risk (up to 8 times) of developing this tumour than the general population.

D. Superficial parotidectomy.

Q6.5
The 60-year-old Chinese lady had a lesion on the anterior surface of the tongue.

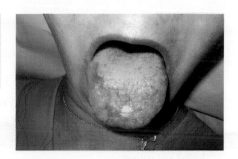

A. What is this condition called?

B. Define the condition.

C. What is the natural history of the condition?

D. What are the risk factors?

E. How would you manage this condition?

Q6.6
This man had a lump in his left neck, which had been growing for the past 3 years.

A. What can be seen in picture A?

B. Which organ could this arise from?

C. What are the differential diagnoses of this swelling?

D. What can be seen in picture B?

E. What are the complications relating to the surgery?

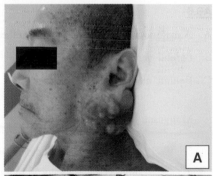

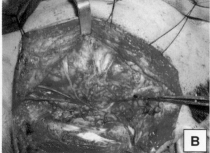

Answers

A6.5

A. Leukoplakia.

B. The World Health Organization (WHO) has defined it as "any white patch or plaque that cannot be characterised clinically or pathologically as any other disease."

C. There is potential for malignant change and the incidence increases with age of the lesion and patient.

D. Tobacco smoking or chewing betel nuts or "lime." There is a weak association with alcohol.

E. Cessation of risk factors is critical as most cases will disappear with removal of them. Any suspicious lesions need histological examination. Regular follow-up is essential.

A6.6

A. A multi-lobulated mass arising from the angle of the jaw lifting the ear lobe.

B. Parotid gland.

C. Benign: pleomorphic adenoma
　　　　　 monomorphic adenoma

　　Malignant: low grade – acinic cell
　　　　　　　　　　　　　 adenoid cystic
　　　　　　　　　　　　　 mucoepidermoid

　　　　　 high grade – adenocarcinoma
　　　　　　　　　　　　 mucoepidermoid

D. Superficial parotidectomy with preservation of the facial nerve.

E. Facial nerve injury, anaesthesia over the ear lobe and Frey's Syndrome. Frey's Syndrome is gustatory sweating of the face and auriculotemporal region due to the regeneration of post-ganglionic secretomotor parasympathetic fibres into the skin.

Q6.7
This patient had previous treatment for oral cancer.

A. What can be seen in picture A and what is the most likely diagnosis?

B. How may we confirm the diagnosis?

C. Which procedure was performed in picture B?

D. Which structures would be sacrificed in this procedure?

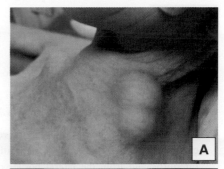

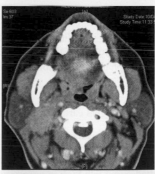

Q6.8
This is a 40-year-old Chinese man who presented with swelling in the right neck.

A. What anomaly can be seen in the CT scans?

B. What is the diagnosis?

C. How else could this patient have presented?

D. What are the aetiological factors?

E. How do we manage the condition?

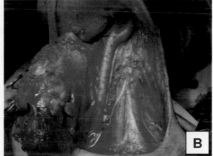

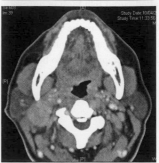

Answers

A6.7

A. Well-circumscribed masses in the left posterior triangle of the neck. Metastases to the cervical lymph nodes.

B. Fine needle aspiration and cytology (FNAC).

C. Radical neck dissection. It refers to the removal of all lymph node groups (level 1–5) extending from the inferior border of the mandible superiorly to the clavicle inferiorly, and from the lateral border of the sternohyoid muscle, hyoid bone and anterior belly of the digastric muscle medially to the anterior border of the trapezius laterally (take reference from the exposed carotid artery).

D. Sternocledomastoid muscle, internal jugular vein and the spinal accessory nerve.

A6.8

A. There is a mass in the right side of the neck deep to the parotid gland and posterior to the mandible. There is fullness in the left nasopharyngeal region (fossa of Rossenmuller).

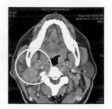

B. Nasopharyngeal carcinoma (NPC) with spread to the lymph nodes.

C. Epistaxis, Otitis media/hearing loss, nasal congestion and cervical lymphadenopathy.

D. Ebstein-Barr virus (EBV) and smoking. Dietary risk factors such as consumption of salted-cured fish high in nitrosamines may play a role in endemic areas of Asia.

E. Radiotherapy is the mainstay of treatment. Surgical treatment is not recommended due to the anatomical constraints in the nasopharynx. Combination therapy with chemotherapy seems to be beneficial for late-stage disease.

Q6.9
This is a 70-year-old Chinese man who presented with difficulty in breathing.

A. What can be seen, based on the picture of the patient?

B. What is the most likely diagnosis?

C. How might the patient have presented?

D. How should the patient be managed?

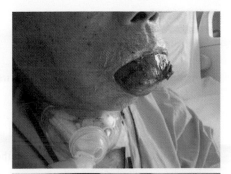

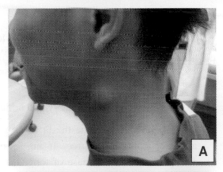

Q6.10
This is a 30-year-old man who had an enlarged neck lymph node.

A. What abnormality can be seen in picture A?

B. What clinical examination should be done?

C. What kind of investigation was performed in picture B?

D. What other investigation should be done?

E. If the investigation above revealed squamous cell carcinoma, what should be done?

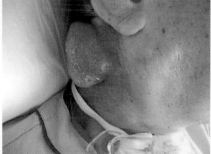

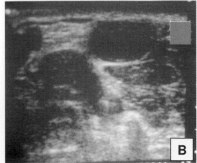

Answers

A6.9

A. a) Mass arising from the right posterior triangle of the neck.
    b) large swollen tongue.
    c) tracheostomy tube.

B. Carcinoma of the tongue that has spread to the cervical lymph nodes.

C. Upper airway obstruction necessitating the tracheostomy.

D. This cancer is in a late stage. The mainstay of treatment would be palliative radiotherapy, ensuring that the airway is not compromised.

A6.10

A. A 3 x 3 cm well-circumscribed circular lesion in the middle third of his left neck.

B. A complete head and neck examination, including the oral cavity.

C. An ultrasound of the neck.

D. Fine needle aspiration of the lymph node.

E. Examination under anaesthesia (EUA) of the mouth, pharynx, larynx, oesophagus and tracheobronchial tree. If no lesion is seen, multiple blind biopsies of the nasopharynx, tonsils, base of tongue, and pyriform sinuses should be performed in the same sitting.

Q6.11
This is a 52-year-old Chinese lady who presented with cervical lymphadenopathy.

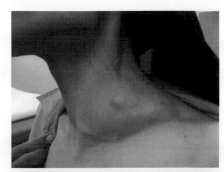

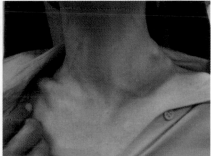

A. Where is the anatomical location of the enlarged lymph nodes?

B. Where are the other levels of lymph nodes in the neck?

C. What are the causes of cervical lymphadenopathy?

Q6.12
This is a 56-year-old man who presented with fever and tender swelling over the left side of the face. Pain on the left jaw was experienced with mastication.

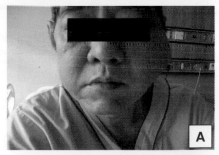

A. What are the differential diagnoses?

B. What other clinical examination would you perform?

C. What investigations would you perform?

D. What investigation is being performed in picture B?

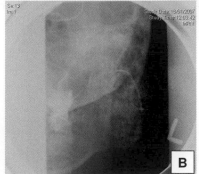

Answers

A6.11

A. The posterior triangle of the neck, level V.

B. level I: submental and submandibular
level II: upper third of the internal jugular vein (IJV)
level III: middle third of IJV
level IV: lower third of IJV
level VI: pre-tracheal

C. **Infection**: Acute (infections of the aerodigestive tract, infectious mononucleosis, toxoplasmosis) and chronic (tuberculosis, sarcoidosis),

Malignancies:

Primary – lymphoma.

Secondary – from the aerodigestive tract or epithelial tumours of the head and neck. (90% of cases are from the head and neck)

A6.12

A. Parotid or masseter abscess, parotid calculi, sialadenitis, mumps or part of a systemic problem (e.g. starvation, bulimia, liver cirrhosis, hypothyroidism).

B. Intra-oral examination.

C. Plain X-ray, ultrasound, sialogram, CT scan
(this patient had a masseter abscess that was drained.)

D. A sialogram.

Q6.13
This patient presented with a neck mass on the right side.

A. What are the findings, based on these investigations?

B. Where does the pathology arise from?

C. Who are at risk?

D. How do they present?

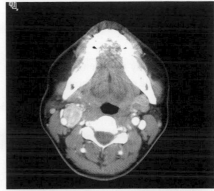

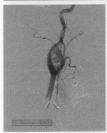
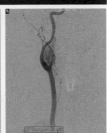

Q6.14
This is a 60-year-old man who had previous surgery.

A. What can be seen in the pictures?

B. What is the diagnosis?

C. What might it be caused by?

D. How else might he present?

E. What are the options to manage the condition?

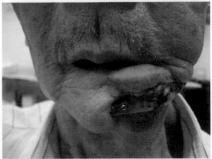

Answers

A6.13

A. Carotid body tumour (classic splaying of the carotid bifurcation with a blush that outlines the normal tumour vessels).

B. It is a rare tumour arising from the chemoreceptor cells on the medial side of the carotid body bulb.

C. High incidence rates for people who reside in high altitudes, those in the 5th decade of their life and those with a family history (10%).

D. Long history of slow-growing painless lump in the neck. The mass is firm, pulsatile and mobile side to side but not up and down.

A6.14

A. Exposure of an implant and the mandible.

B. Osteoradionecrosis.

C. Non-vital bone secondary to radiation injury. There is absence of reserve reparative capacity.

D. Pain, swelling, trismus, malocclusion, oral cutaneous fistula and pathological fractures.

E. Medical therapy is mainly supportive. Hyperbaric oxygen has been shown to be useful. Surgical options for closure of the wound include microvascular free tissue transfer.

Chapter 7

BREAST

Q7.1
The 56-year-old lady had a left breast lump that had increased in size over 6 months.

A. What is a "triple assessment"?

B. Which investigations are being carried out in the pictures?

C. Describe the features in the left breast.

D. What procedures can you carry out in the clinic to further evaluate the breast lump?

E. What is the management mode of this patient?

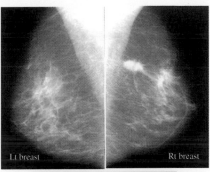

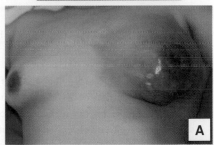

Q7.2
The 45-year-old woman presented with a mass in the left breast.

A. Describe the findings in picture A.

B. What are the possible differential diagnoses?

C. What are the important aspects of the patient's history?

D. Which is the best way to make a diagnosis?

E. What investigations are done to stage the disease?

F. What procedure has been performed in picture B and what can be seen?

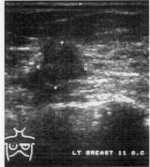

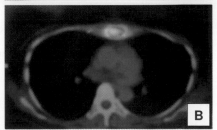

Answers

A7.1

A. It is obtaining a diagnosis through the combined assessment of a breast lump from clinical, radiological and pathological examination.

B. Bilateral mammogram and ultrasound.

C. Distortion of the breast parenchyma with calcifications.

D. Fine needle aspiration and cytology (FNAC) or core biopsy.

E. Confirmation of a cancer and stage the disease.

A7.2

A. There is a large, lobulated ulcerating, inflammed mass in the left breast.

B. Breast carcinoma or abscess.

C. The length of time since the onset of the lump (enlarging or reducing) and any associated tenderness or fever. Others include risk factors for breast cancer; the age at menarche, family history of breast cancer, number of children, age at childbirth and drug history (oral contraceptive pill/hormone replacement therapy).

D. Obtain a histological/cytological biopsy (this patient had a carcinoma).

E. Chest X-ray, liver ultrasound and bone scan.

F. Positron emission tomography (PET) showing metastatic spread to the sternum.

Q7.3
The 55-year-old lady had a mastectomy.

A. What can be seen in the macroscopic specimen?

B. What can be seen in the histological specimen?

C. What are predictors of poor outcome?

D. What molecular markers are currently available and how do they influence prognosis?

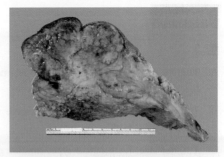

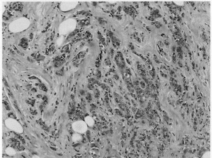

Q7.4
This 45-year-old lady had needle localisation and excision of a breast lesion.

A. What can be seen in picture A?

B. What can be seen in picture B and what is the diagnosis?

C. What are the implications of the diagnosis?

D. Who are most at risk and how does this condition present?

E. How are patients with this condition managed?

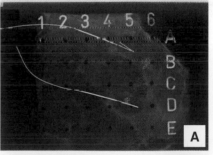

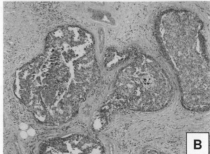

Answers

A7.3

A. The cut surface of a mastectomy specimen showing a large infiltrative solid tumour mass with involvement of the skin.

B. The tumour is composed of infiltrative malignant cells disposed in cord and nests, lying within fibroblastic stroma.

C. Tumour size, histological type, tumour grade, nodal involvement, vascular invasion and multicentricity, tumour- involved excision margins.

D. Oestrogen and Progesterone receptors (ER and PR) – ER/PR positive tumours have a good response rate to chemotherapy compared to ER/PR negative tumours.

ERBB-2 (HER2) positivity – a humanised anti-ERBB-2 monoclonal antibody trastuzumab (Herceptin) is effective in some patients with over expression of ERBB-2.

A7.4

A. The patient had areas of microcalcification (5B and 5C) in the breast tissue. This is radiological confirmation that the suspicious lesion has been excised.

B. Tumour cells are seen within ducts and confined to the basement membrane. Ductal Carcinoma In Situ (DCIS).

C. It is a pre-invasive carcinomatous process. If left untreated, it often proceeds to invasive ductal carcinoma. There is a 25–50% risk of breast cancer in 10–15 years.

D. It affects patients predominantly between 40 to 60 years of age, and often presents as suspicious microcalcifications on mammography or with nipple discharge and/or mass.

E. **Localised (<4 cm) lesions** are treated by wide local excision +/− radiotherapy and tamoxifen.

Widespread/multifocal lesions are treated by mastectomy +/− tamoxifen.

Q7.5
A 25-year-old girl presented with a mobile breast lump that was excised.

A. What are the differential diagnoses of breast lumps for patients in this age group?

B. What is the probable diagnosis?

C. How does it present?

D. What can be seen from the histology specimen?

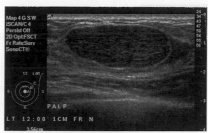

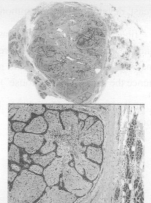

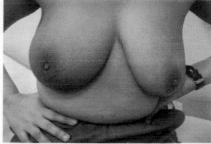

Q7.6
A 40-year-old lady presented with "heaviness" and associated skin changes in her right breast.

A. Describe the abnormal physical signs that can be seen in the pictures.

B. List two conditions that can give rise to the above appearance.

C. What is the pathogenesis?

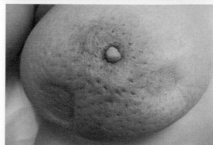

Answers

A7.5

A. Fibroadenomas are common in young women. Breast cysts are common for women between 30 to 50 years of age. New lumps in women above 50 years of age should be investigated for a carcinoma until proven otherwise.

B. Fibroadenoma of the breast. It is the most common benign tumour of the female breast, developing most commonly during the reproductive period of a woman.

C. A fibroadenoma presents as a well-circumscribed palpable mass, ovoid mammographic density or well- circumscribed smooth lesions on ultrasound imaging. It is often mobile and may disappear from between the fingers on palpation (hence the term, "breast mouse").

D. A well-circumscribed biphasic lesion consisting of benign stroma and epithelium-lined cystic spaces.

A7.6

A. Enlarged right breast with "peau d'orange" appearance of the right breast.

B. Breast carcinoma or abscess.

C. It is due to cutaneous lymphatic oedema. The infiltrated skin is tethered to the sweat ducts and subsequently cannot swell, giving the appearance of tiny pits resembling that of orange peel.

Q7.7
A 40-year-old lady experienced pain in her left breast.

A. What abnormality can be seen in picture A?

B. What is the most likely diagnosis?

C. What can be seen from the bone scan in picture B?

D. How can we manage the patient?

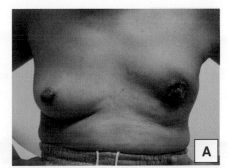

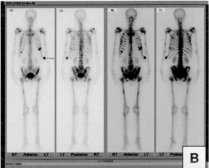

Q7.8
A 50-year-old lady presented with swelling and ulceration of her right breast for 2 years.

A. What is the most likely diagnosis and how would you confirm it?

B. What is the first-line treatment for this patient?

C. What is the most useful receptor marker of this disease and what drug can be added if this receptor is present?

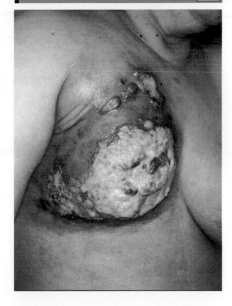

Answers

A7.7

A. There is an ulcerated lesion that involves the left nipple and has eroded into the left breast.

B. Invasive breast carcinoma.

C. Evidence of multiple bone metastases.

D. This patient has metastatic disease. She will require palliative systemic therapy to alleviate symptoms. Hormone manipulation is often the first-line treatment because of its minimal side effects. Local radiotherapy can be useful for painful bony deposits.

A7.8

A. It is most likely a breast carcinoma and a biopsy (FNA, core or wedge incision) can be done to confirm it.

B. Neo-adjuvant therapy, chemotherapy or radiotherapy (the intention is to "shrink" the tumour to facilitate a less morbid toilet mastectomy as adequate skin closure is a concern).

C. The cytosol of breast cancer cells may contain oestrogen (ER) and progesterone (PR) receptors. ER activity is present in 60% and represents a biochemical marker for the degree of differentiation and histological subtype. ER positive tumours have a better response to hormonal manipulation. Tamoxifen is a triphenylamine anti-oestrogen that blocks the effect of endogenous oestrogen. Approximately 30% of all breast cancers respond to tamoxifen. This rises to 60% if they are ER-positive.

Q7.9
A 35-year-old woman presented with a right nipple discharge for a duration of 1 month.

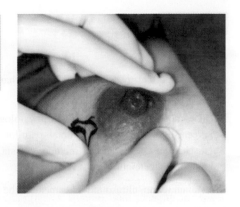

A. What other information about the discharge is important?

B. What are the common causes of this kind of nipple discharge?

C. Which kinds of non-invasive investigations would you perform to help manage the condition?

D. If the investigations are not conclusive and the nipple discharge persists, what else can you do?

Q7.10
This lady had a procedure performed after routine breast screening.

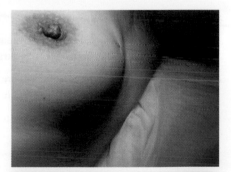

A. Which procedure has been performed on this patient, based on the pictures?

B. How may these lesions present?

C. What is done immediately after the excision of the breast tissue?

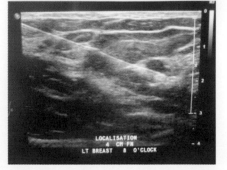

Answers

A7.9

A. It is important to determine if the discharge is from a single or multiple duct, and whether it is unilateral or bilateral.

B. The most common cause is a physiological discharge that varies from clear to greenish brown. An intraductal papilloma presents as a unilateral blood stained discharge. Other causes include ectasia, papillomatosis and prolactinomas. An intraductal carcinoma must be ruled out.

C. Mammogram, ultrasound and smear of the discharge for cytology and culture.

D. Microdochectomy/excision of duct system; duct lavage and cytological examination.

A7.10

A. Radiological needle localisation of a breast lesion that is diagnosed to be abnormal or suspicious, either on mammogram or ultrasound scans.

B. They are generally asymptomatic and are diagnosed either during screening or during investigation for another unrelated problem.

C. It is sent for radiological examination to confirm that the localised lesion has been completely removed.

Q7.11
This lady had surgery in her left axilla.

A. What kind of surgery was performed?

B. What is the rationale for the surgery?

C. Why is it important in breast surgery?

D. How is it isolated?

E. In what other pathologies is this mode of surgery used?

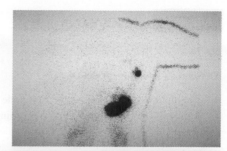

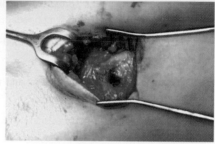

Q7.12
The 48-year-old lady recently noticed that her left breast looked different.

A. What abnormality can you observe?

B. What may be the cause?

C. What problems might the patient encounter?

D. What diagnostic tests would you order for this patient?

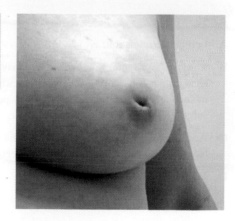

Answers

A7.11

A. Sentinel lymph node biopsy.

B. The sentinel lymph node is the first node that drains into the lymphatic basin. If it is not involved with a tumour, the remaining lymph nodes will assumed to be clear of disease.

C. If there is no tumour spread to the node, an axillary clearance, which may be associated with upper limb lymphoedema, can be avoided.

D. Injected blue dye or technetium-labeled sulphur colloid injected either periareolar or into the tumour.

E. Management of penile carcinomas and malignant melanomas to determine the need for regional lymphadenectomy.

A7.12

A. Left nipple retraction.

B. It may be congenital where the nipple may evert at any time as the breast develops or changes, such as during pregnancy or when it undergoes involution. Other causes include carcinoma, mammary fistula, periductal fibrosis, duct ectasia, previous surgery, chronic abscess, Paget's Disease.

C. Apart from the aesthetic concern, she might have difficulty breastfeeding and may have an increased risk of developing infections.

D. Mammogram and ultrasound.

Q7.13
This 25-year-old lady was 3 months post-partum. She had undergone emergency breast surgery.

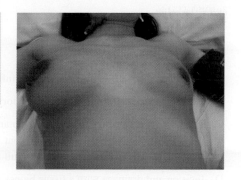

A. What abnormality can be seen in this patient?

B. What is the differential diagnosis?

C. Who are more susceptible to this condition?

D. How should the condition be managed?

Q7.14
This is a 52-year-old Chinese lady who had surgery.

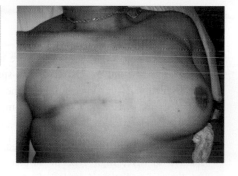

A. What surgery was performed?

B. What are the variations of this surgery?

C. What are its indications?

D. What are the options for reconstruction?

Answers

A7.13

A. An enlarged right breast that is red and inflamed.

B. Breast abscess, cellulitis, and inflammatory breast cancer.

C. The first group belongs to mothers who are breastfeeding. The second group belongs to patients who have a history of recent trauma (e.g. jogger's nipple). The painful swelling is usually accompanied by a dull ache but progresses to a throbbing pain.

D. Incision and drainage with a tissue biopsy (to exclude a carcinoma).

A7.14

A. Total right mastectomy.

B. **Subcutaneous** (all the breast tissue are removed except for the overlying skin and nipple-areolar complex (NAC)), **skin-sparing** (all the breast tissue are removed except for overlying skin), **total** (all the breast tissue, overlying skin and NAC are removed) and **radical** (a total mastectomy with pectoralis muscle and axillary lymph nodes removed).

C. **Therapeutic**: carcinoma – widespread DCIS, subareolar tumour, large tumour relative to size, high risk of further disease (BRCA -1/-2 positive), previous irradiation, irradiation is contraindicated and patient preference.

   Prophylactic: strong family history of breast cancer.

D. All should be offered reconstruction; prosthetic or autologous; immediate or delayed to create a new breast mound.

Chapter **8**

UPPER GI

Q8.1
This is an endoscopic view of the oesophagus.

A. What can be seen in picture A?

B. How may this present clinically?

C. What are the possible causes?

D. Which procedure was performed, based on pictures B and C?

E. What are the potential complications of the procedure?

F. What adjunctive procedure might be carried out in picture E so as to augment the previous procedure?

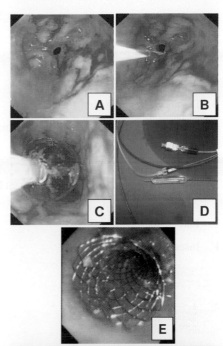

Q8.2
A 20-year-old man presented with worsening dysphagia, regurgitation and chest pain.

A. What investigation was performed?

B. What is the radiological appearance and diagnosis?

C. What is the definition of this disorder?

D. What other investigation can be done to confirm the disorder?

E. How may this condition be treated?

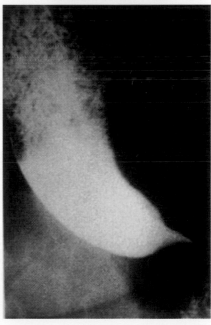

Answers

A8.1

A. Narrowing/stricture of the oesophagus.

B. Dysphagia, regurgitation and vomiting.

C. Benign: long-standing reflux disease, anastomotic strictures and ingestion of caustic agents.

Malignant: Carcinoma.

D. Insertion of a guide wire and subsequent balloon dilatation of the esophagus.

E. Early: bleeding and perforation.
Late: re-narrowing.

F. Insertion of a stent.

A8.2

A. Barium swallow.

B. Dilatation of the proximal oesophagus with a "beak-like" tapering distally is highly suggestive of achalasia.

C. It is the most common primary oesophageal motility disorder caused by inflammation of the myenteric plexus, leading to fibrosis with decrease and loss of myenteric ganglion cells.

D. Manometric studies would reveal absence of peristaltic contractions and incomplete relaxation and abnormally high pressures of the lower oesophageal sphincter.

E. Botulinum toxin injection provides temporary relief and symptomatic improvement. Pneumatic dilatation is more effective but is associated with recurrence within 5 years.

Surgical myotomy (Heller's cardiomyotomy) is considered after failure of the previous non-surgical treatments, younger patients and when there is other co-existing pathology requiring surgical intervention.

Q8.3
This is a specimen removed en bloc from a man who had a tumour in the stomach.

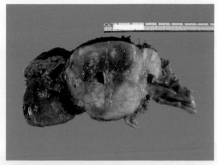

A. In the picture showing the gross specimen, which organ was resected with the stomach?

B. What can be seen in the microscopic specimen?

C. What kind of tumour is this and where do they originate from?

D. What is the diagnostic criterion?

E. What determines its malignant potential?

F. What adjuvant treatment may be useful?

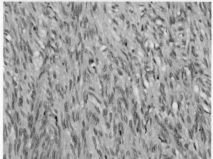

Q8.4
This scan is of a 45-year-old man who presented with vague upper abdominal discomfort.

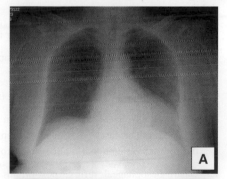

A. What can be seen in picture A?

B. What investigation was carried in picture B and what does it show?

C. What is the diagnosis and what types are there?

D. What is the pathogenesis?

E. What symptoms would the patient complain of?

F. What are the possible complications?

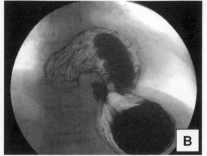

Answers

A8.3

A. The spleen.

B. Predominent spindle cell proliferation with absence of epithelial cells.

C. It is an uncommon tumour of the gastrointestinal tract. They arise from the mesenchymal layer from the Cajal (pacemaker cells of the gastrointestinal tract) cells. 70% occur in the stomach and 20% in the small intestine and the rest, elsewhere in the gastrointestinal tract.

D. By histopathology with positive immunohistochemical staining for c-kit (CD117) (tyrosine kinase).

E. This size of the tumour and mitotic rate of tumour cells.

F. Tyrosine kinse inhibitors (e.g. Imatinib).

A8.4

A. An air fluid level is seen in the posterior mediastinum on the chest X-ray.

B. The barium swallow shows the upper part of the stomach herniating through a tear or weakness in the diaphragm.

C. Hiatus hernia. The types include sliding (more common) and para-oesophageal.

D. The distal esophagus is normally held in position by a fusion of the endothoracic and endoabdominal fascia at the diaphragmatic hiatus called the phreno-oesophageal membrane. Weakness of it allows the protrusion of the stomach.

E. Gastro-oesophageal reflux, post-prandial pain, early satiety, breathlessness with meals and dysphagia.

F. A herniated gastric pouch is susceptible to volvulus, obstruction, bleeding and infection.

Q8.5
This is the barium swallow study of a 70-year-old male who presented with dysphagia.

A. What does the picture reveal?

B. What is the most likely diagnosis?

C. Which kind of additional investigation would be useful?

D. What is the alternative to surgical treatment?

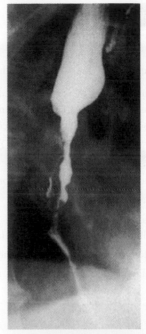

Q8.6
This man presented with progressive dysphagia and was initially treated with neoadjuvant chemo-radiotherapy.

A. Describe the abnormal endoscopic findings in picture A.

B. What is your diagnosis?

C. What kind of investigation was performed in picture B. Why was it carried out?

D. What is the most likely histological type?

E. What is neoadjuvant therapy and what are its advantages and disadvantages?

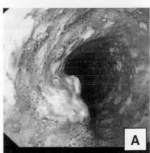

Mid Esophagus

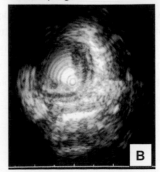

Answers

A8.5

A. Narrowing of the esophagus with shouldering.

B. Carcinoma of the oesophagus. Most oesophageal carcinomas fall into one of two classes: squamous cell carcinoma, which are similar to head and neck cancers and associated with tobacco and alcohol consumption, and adenocarcinomas, which are associated with having a history of gastro-oesophageal reflux disease and Barrett's oesophagus.

C. Endoscopic ultrasound, CT thorax and liver ultrasound may be used to stage the disease.

D. Radiotherapy – super voltage external beam radiotherapy may be curative or palliative to relieve dysphagia. Brachytherapy may be another option.

Chemotherapy – most regimes have 5FU with or without leucovorin.

Palliation to relieve dysphagia – re-canalisation or intubation with a stent.

A8.6

A. There is a ulcerated irregular mass arising from the oesophagus.

B. Carcinoma of the oesophagus.

C. Endoscopic ultrasound (EUS) helps to determine **T** stage of disease (depth of the Tumour growth) which influences choice of management between surgery and chemo radiation.

D. Squamous cell carcinoma (upper 2/3) and adenocarcinoma (lower 1/3).

E. Treatment with chemotherapy and/or radiation to the primary lesion before surgery.

Advantages: There is potential down-staging (to shrink the tumour), early treatment of micrometastatic disease, treatment is better tolerated before surgical stress and verification of the tumours sensitivity to this particular therapy.

Disadvantages: Delay in the treatment of the primary lesion, selection for chemoresistent cell lines and potentially cause the tissue around the tumour to be inflammed or fibrosed.

Q8.7
This 50-year-old man presented with progressive dysphagia.

A. What can be seen in picture A?

B. What is shown in picture B?

C. What surgery did the patient undergo?

D. Which other organ may be used as a conduit for the reconstruction of gastrointestinal continuity?

E. What are the risks of this surgery?

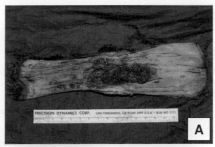

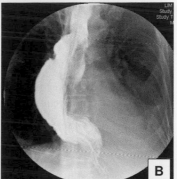

Q8.8
An emergency gastroscopy was performed on this patient.

A. What can be seen in picture A?

B. How would the patient have presented?

C. What would have been subsequently done during the endoscopy shown in picture B?

D. If bleeding is controlled, how would the patient be managed?

E. What should be done if bleeding continues?

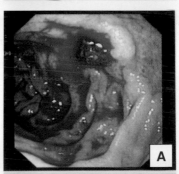

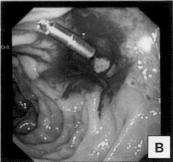

Answers

A8.7

A. A resected specimen of an oesophageal tumour with adequate macroscopic proximal and distal margins.

B. Radiological evidence of a gastric pull-up in the mediastinum.

C. Ivor Lewis oesophagectomy with oesophago-gastric anastomosis in the right chest.

  Other areas of anastomosis include the neck or abdomen; depending on the site of tumour; and the length of the oesophagus to be resected; for proximal and distal clearance.

D. Free colon interposition.

E. This surgery is associated with high morbidity. Complications include haemorrhage, anastomotic leak, empyema, chyle leak, chest infection and anastomotic stricture.

A8.8

A. Oozing from an exposed vessel in the duodenum.

B. Haematemesis or malaena and hypovolaemic shock.

C. Attempted haemostasis with endoclips. Other various methods include adrenaline injection and thermal coagulation.

D. Start the patient on intravenous anti-acid therapy (with a proton pump inhibitor) and monitor closely for re-bleeding.

E. Resuscitate and arrange for immediate surgery. This is often an under-running of the ulcer with the option of an acid reducing procedure (vagotomy).

Q8.9
The 60-year-old man had suffered a stroke.

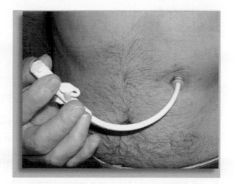

A. What can be seen in this picture?

B. How is the equipment inserted?

C. Why would a patient need the equipment?

D. What complications may develop during its usage?

E. What are the alternatives to the tube?

Q8.10
This obese 40-year-old man underwent surgery.

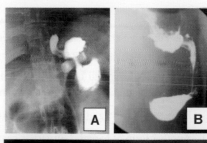

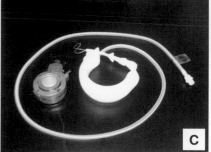

A. What can be seen in picture A and what kind of surgery was performed using the prosthesis in picture C?

B. What are the indications for this procedure?

C. How is BMI calculated?

D. Name an alternative operative procedure as seen in the post-operative radiological study in picture B?

E. What are the medical conditions associated with this body habitus?

Answers

A8.9

A. A gastrostomy tube.

B. Percutanous Endoscopic Gastrostomy (PEG) or open method.

C. It is used for enteral feeding when per-oral feeding cannot be carried out due to a mechanical obstruction or a neurological cause affecting the swallowing mechanism.

D. Blockade or dislodgement of the tube, which requires a replacement.

E. A nasogastric tube or a jejunostomy tube.

A8.10

A. The radiological study shows a contracted stomach with a gastric band across it. The prosthesis used is seen in picture C.

B. Patients with morbid obesity (elevated Body Mass Index) who have failed to lose weight with dietary modification and pharmacological treatment.

C. Body weight (in kg) divided by height (in metres) squared.

D. Another form of bariatric surgery is gastric bypass (malabsorptive) surgery.

E. Sleep apnea, coronary artery disease, pulmonary disease, diabetes, arthritis and so forth.

Q8.11
A 51-year-old man presented with a 6 months history of anorexia, pallor and weight loss.

A. What can be seen in the gross specimen and what surgical procedure had been performed?

B. What can be observed in the microscopic specimen?

C. What are the two types of adenocarcinoma?

D. What are the aetiological factors of this pathological condition?

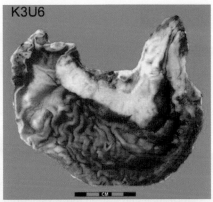
K3U6

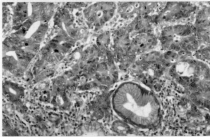

Q8.12
The 36-year-old man was a chronic heavy smoker and presented with early satiety.

A. What can be observed in these pictures?

B. What is characteristic of the vomiting relating to this pathology?

C. What might you find when examining the abdomen?

D. What needs to be performed during endoscopy and how would the patient be managed?

E. If the biopsy result is "active gastritis," what should be done next?

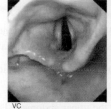
VC

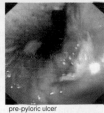
pre-pyloric ulcer

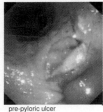
pre-pyloric ulcer

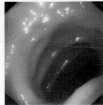
duodenum

Answers

A8.11

A. There is a tumour in the lesser curve of the stomach. A total gastrectomy was performed.

B. Normal columnar epithelium is replaced by poorly differentiated adenocarcinoma exhibiting an infiltrative growth pattern.

C. Intestinal type – commoner, polypoid masses, has gland formation with intraglandular mucin, ulcerates and is associated with a better prognosis.

Diffuse type – spreads through the wall, "leatherbottle stomach," has no gland formation and instead forms signet-ring cells with intracellular mucin.

D. Environment: Diet (lack of fruit and vegetables), cigarette smoking.

Host: infection by *Helicobacter Pylori*, leading to chronic gastritis, autoimmune gastritis, partial gastrectomy.

Dysplasia is the final common pathway.

A8.12

A. A pre-pyloric gastric ulcer with evidence of gastric outlet obstruction (there should not be food debris after these patients have fasted for more than 6 hours).

B. The vomiting is projectile and the vomitus is characterised by an absence of bile and the presence of partially digested food.

C. A mass arising in the upper abdomen. This "mass" is a distended stomach. If it is full of food, it will be a firm mass which is dull to percussion. If there is air and fluid, a succussion splash can be elicited.

D. A biopsy to exclude a cancer as a cause for the ulcer, check for urease activity and start acid suppression medication.

E. Repeat a gastroscopy to look for healing of the ulcer and repeat the biopsy if it remains the same.

Q8.13
This is a specimen of a 40-year-old man who presented with iron-deficiency anaemia.

A. What is the diagnosis?

B. What are the possible histological types?

C. What surgery was performed?

D. What is the clinical use of lymph node dissection?

E. What are the possible post-operative complications specific to the surgery?

F. What can be seen in the endoscopic pictures?

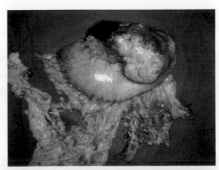

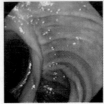

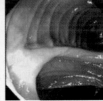

Roux loop 85cm

Roux loop 85cm

Q8.14
This is an endoscopic view of the lower oesophagus in 2 different patients.

A. What can be seen in picture A?

B. What can be seen in picture B and what is the diagnosis?

C. What symptoms might the patient in picture B have?

D. What is the pathogenesis?

E. How should this condition be managed?

F. What percentage of patients fail conservative therapy and how can they be managed?

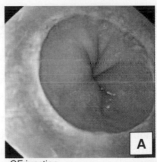

GE junction

A

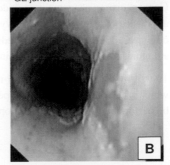

B

Answers

A8.13

A. Gastric cancer. It is the fourth most common cancer worldwide and the second most common cause of cancer death worldwide after lung cancer.

B. Adenocarcinoma (most common), lymphoma, Gastrointestinal stromal tumours.

C. D2 lymphadenectomy and gastrectomy (level 1 and 2 lymph nodes as seen by the omentectomy).

D. It provides better accuracy for staging and offer radical local clearance. Some studies have shown improved survival in patients with stage 2 and 3a disease.

E. Dumping syndrome – early and late, alkaline reflux gastritis, roux stasis syndrome, loop syndromes (efferent and afferent), post-vagotomy diarrhoea, nutritional deficiencies (iron, folate, vitamin B12 and calcium).

F. The roux-loop anastomosis between the stomach and jejunum after the subtotal gastrectomy.

A8.14

A. A normal gastro-oesophageal junction.

B. There are superficial mucosal erosions and ulcerations. Reflux oesophagitis.

C. Heartburn dysphagia and acid regurgitation. The discomfort is often relieved by antacids. The DeMeester scoring system is useful for assessing severity.

D. The factors include: weakness of the lower oesophageal sphincter (LOS), short length of intra-abdominal segment of oesophagus, inappropriate LOS relaxations, delayed gastric emptying and hiatus hernia.

E. Conservative management includes the cessation of smoking and alcohol intake, avoidance of spicy food and heavy meals prior to bedtime, weight loss and elevating one's head when in bed. Medications include antacids, histamine-2-receptors antagonists and proton pump inibitors (PPI).

F. 10–15% will be referred for anti-reflux surgery. It is a fundoplication procedure in which the gastric fundus is wrapped around the lower end of the oesophagus. It can be performed by laparoscopic or open surgery.

Chapter 9

UROLOGY

Q9.1
**A 55-year-old male complained of left loin pain and fever.
On examination, he was found to have a palpable left-sided abdominal mass.**

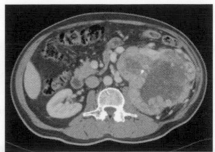

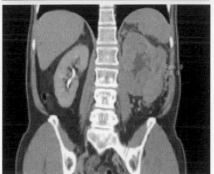

A. What is the diagnosis?

B. What is the most common histological cell type?

C. How do they present?

D. What should you look out for during the CT scan?

E. How can we manage this patient?

Q9.2
This patient underwent a nephrectomy.

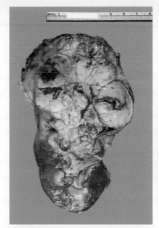

A. What is the most likely diagnosis?

B. What can be seen macroscopically?

C. What are the risk factors?

D. Which group of individuals is most at risk?

E. What genetic condition predisposes one to it?

F. What can be seen microscopically?

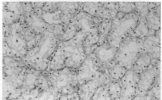

Answers

A9.1

A. Renal cell carcinoma (hypernephroma or Grawitz's tumour). It is the most common form of kidney cancer.

B. Seventy-five per cent are adenocarcinoma and they arise from the proximal tubular cells.

C. A classic triad is often described. It includes haematuria with or without clot colic; occurring in 90% of patients, dragging discomfort in the loin and an abdominal mass. Other presentations include varicocele, persistent pyrexia or para-neoplastic syndromes.

D. Size of the mass, invasion into adjacent structures, presence of enlarged lymph nodes and involvement of the renal vein and inferior vena cava.

E. Radical surgery offers the best chance. The en bloc resection involves the removal of the kidney, upper ureters, renal vessels, adrenal glands and Gerota's fascia.

A9.2

A. Renal cell carcinoma.

B. These tumours appear as a spherical mass composed of bright yellow-grey-white tissue that distorts the renal outline. There are also areas of necrosis, foci of haemorrhagic discolouration and areas of softening.

C. Smoking is the most important factor. There are weak associations with high dietary consumption of fats and oil, and exposure to toxic agents (lead, cadmium, asbestos).

D. Males in their 50–60s.

E. Von Hippel-Lindau (VHL) Syndrome.

F. They are cells with clear or granular cytoplasm arranged in nests and tubules, which give rise to their name, clear cell carcinoma.

Q9.3
This 60-year-old man presented with a lump in the penis.

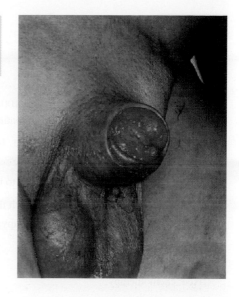

A. What is the abnormality?

B. How common is this condition and who are usually affected?

C. What are the associated factors?

D. What is the cell type and where does it spread to?

E. How should this condition be managed?

Q9.4
The 30-year-old man complained of a mass in his left scrotum.

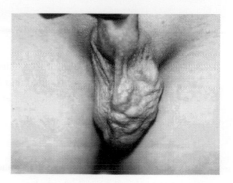

A. What abnormality can be seen?

B. What is the pathology?

C. How may this condition present?

D. What is the classical description of the condition upon examination in a standing position?

E. How should the condition be managed?

F. It this condition was of recent onset and the mass does not empty when in a supine position, what is your concern?

Answers

A9.3

A. Cancer of the penis.

B. It is uncommon, occurring one per 100,000 males. It is common in those over 60 years of age and rarely develops in patients who are circumcised.

C. Long-standing phimosis, poor penile hygiene, human papilloma virus (HPV) infection, smoking and oriental ethnicity.

D. Squamous cell carcinoma. They spread to the inguinal lymph nodes.

E. **(Penis)** It depends on the extent to which the penis is affected.

   prepuce: circumcision; glans: radiotherapy; shaft: partial or total amputation.

   (metastatic inguinal lymph nodes)

   mobile: en bloc resection;
   fixed: chemotherapy.

A9.4

A. Left-sided varicocele.

B. Varicosities of the pampiniform plexus of veins, which drain the testicle. The majority (90%) of cases is left-sided and due to incompetence or absence of the valve at the termination of the left testicular vein before its insertion into the renal vein.

C. A dull ache in the scrotum or infertility.

D. It feels like "a bag of worms."

E. Surgical intervention-ligation of the gonadal veins.

   (low tie): within the inguinal canal.
   (high tie): retroperitoneal above the deep ring.

   An alternative to surgery is radiological embolisation.

F. It may be due to venous occlusion by a renal or retroperitoneal tumour.

Q9.5
A 60-year-old man complained of dribbling when urinating and a sensation of incomplete bladder emptying.

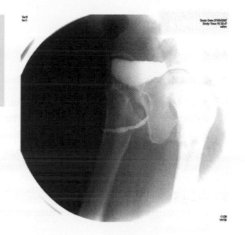

A. What is the radiological study being carried out and what does it reveal?

B. How is it performed?

C. List three causes of this condition.

D. What other symptoms may develop?

E. What is the management mode?

Q9.6
A 60-year-old Chinese man complained of painless haematuria. A flexible cystoscopy was performed.

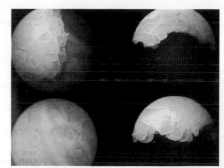

A. What is your diagnosis?

B. Who are most at risk?

C. What are the risk factors?

D. What treatment option can you offer the patient?

E. What can be seen microscopically?

F. What governs prognosis?

G. How should we follow-up the patient?

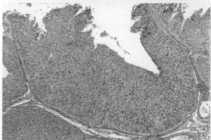

Answers

A9.5

A. Retrograde urethrogram showing a urethral stricture.

B. A 14-French Foley catheter is placed into the urethra without lubrication so that the balloon is 2–3 cm beyond the meatus. The balloon is then inflated with 1–2 cc to seat it in the fossa navicularis. With the patient in 30-degree oblique position, 30 mL of half strength contrast is injected through the catheter. The radiograph is exposed when the contrast is nearly completely injected.

C. Trauma, infection and previous instrumentation.

D. Other obstructive symptoms include urinary intermittency and increased frequency of micturation.

E. Urethral dilation with sound probes, optical urethrotomy or urethroplasty.

A9.6

A. Bladder carcinoma-superficial (Ta,T1).

B. Males are affected by three times. More common in Caucasians than Africans.

C. Smoking, industrial carcinogens (aromatic amines) and schistosomiasis.

D. Transurethral resection of bladder tumour (TURBT).

E. Transitional cell (urothelial) carcinoma featuring thickened neoplastic urothelium with a papillary architecture.

F. Treatment will be performed based on the grade and stage of the disease.

G. Regular cystoscopic examinations. The overall recurrence is 50–60% and the development of invasion is low.

Q9.7
An intravenous urogram was performed on a 60-year-old man.

A. What are the two significant findings, based on the radiological investigation?

B. What can be observed in the gross specimen?

C. How does this condition present?

D. What surgery was performed?

E. What is an alternative to surgery?

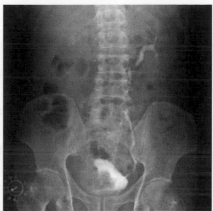

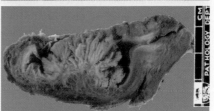

Q9.8
This 45-year-old man suffered from abdominal discomfort.

A. Based on the scans, what is this patient suffering from?

B. How else might he present?

C. What is the prognosis?

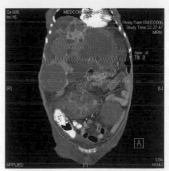

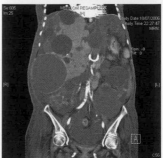

Answers

A9.7

A. Filling defect in the right side of the bladder and delayed opacification of the right kidney.

B. There is a papillary tumour arising from mucosa of the resected bladder.

C. Painless haematuria (gross or microscopic) is the most common symptom. Frequency, urgency and dysuria may also be present.

D. A radical cystectomy with urinary diversion, either as a conduit or a continent reservoir.

E. Radical radiotherapy. It leaves the patient with a bladder and without appliance. This treatment is however associated with radiation cystitis and proctitis. Other treatment options include topical chemotherapy and BCG therapy.

A9.8

A. Polycystic liver and kidney disease. It is a progressive genetic disorder of the kidneys. The two major forms of polycystic kidney disease are distinguished by their patterns of inheritance: autosomal dominant and autosomal recessive.

B. If it affects only the liver, the condition is often asymptomatic. Occasionally it presents with hepatomegaly. If the kidney is affected, it may present with renal enlargement, pain, haematuria, infection and hypertension.

C. Chronic renal failure develops as the functioning renal tissue is slowly replaced by cysts. End-stage renal failure often begins in middle life and the patient is unlikely to survive without renal replacement by dialysis or transplant.

Q9.9
An 16-year-old boy complained of left scrotal pain for 4 hours. A duplex ultrasound of the testis was done.

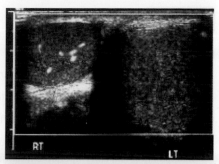

A. What abnormality can be seen in the ultrasound scan?

B. What does the gross specimen show and what is your diagnosis?

C. What would you have found during a clinical examination?

D. What is the management of this condition?

E. What should be done to the contralateral testis?

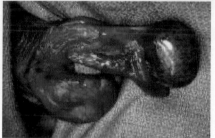

Q9.10
The 52-year-old man presented with increasing scrotal discomfort for 3 months.

A. What can be seen in picture A?

B. What surgical procedure was performed in picture B and what was the approach used?

C. What is your diagnosis if the abnormality was found in a 20-year old?

D. What is the lymphatic spread?

E. How are they staged?

F. What is the prognosis?

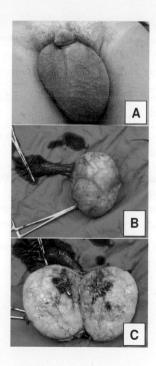

Answers

A9.9

A. Doppler ultrasound confirming the absence of blood supply to the affected left testis.

B. An infarcted testis due to torsion of the testis.

C. There would be a tender, high-riding left testis with an oblique lie.

D. If treatment is administered early, untwisting may be successful with gentle manipulation and early operative fixation to avoid a recurrent torsion.

If diagnosis is uncertain or late, exploration through a scrotal incision is performed:
viable: untwist and orchidopexy.
infarcted: orchidectomy.

E. The other side should be fixed because anatomical variation responsible for the torsion of the ipsilateral side.

A9.10

A. An enlarged left scrotal mass.

B. Radical orchidectomy via the inguinal approach.

C. Seminoma (40% of tumours of the testis). Cut surface is typically homogenous and pink in colour.

D. To the retro-peritoneal and intra-thoracic lymph nodes (not to the inguinal lymph nodes).

E. Stage 1. testis lesion, no nodal involvement.
Stage 2. nodes below diaphragm.
Stage 3. nodes above the diaphragm.
Stage 4. pulmonary and hepatic metastases.

F. No metastases: 5-year survival rate of 95% after orchidectomy and radiotherapy or chemotherapy.

Q9.11
This test was performed on an elderly male patient with urinary symptoms.

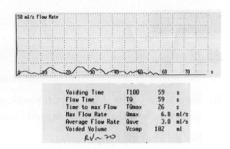

A. What is this test called?

B. What does the result imply?

C. What is the most likely diagnosis?

D. What are the different treatment options available for this condition?

Q9.12
This is a pathological specimen of the patient's lower urinary tract, including the bladder.

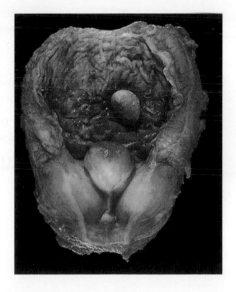

A. What is the pathology, based on the specimen?

B. What investigations should be carried out?

C. What are the indications for treatment?

D. What approaches can be used during surgery?

Answers

A9.11

A. Uroflowmetry and post-void residual urine measurement.

B. Slow urinary flow, low Qmax 6.8 ml/s, prolonged voiding time (59 s), low residual urine volume (20 ml). These suggest bladder outlet obstruction.

C. Benign prostatic hypertrophy.

D. **Medical treatment**: e.g. alpha-adreneric blocker and 5 alpha reductase blockers.

   Surgery: Transurethral resection of the prostate (TURP) is the most common surgical treatment in which the adenomatous portion of the prostate is removed via a rectoscope, using electrocautery from the prostatic urethra.

A9.12

A. Tri-lobar benign prostatic hypertrophy (BPH) with bladder calculus and wall hypertrophy.

B. Urinary symptom score, serum creatinine, urinalysis and culture, uroflowmetry and ultrasound scans of the bladder and kidneys.

C. Acute or chronic retention leading to renal impairment, complications of bladder outflow obstruction (stone, infection and diverticular formation) and haemorrhaging.

D. Trans-urethral (TURP), trans-vesical (TVP), retropubic (RPP) and through the perineum.

Q9.13
The 80-year-old Chinese man complained of worsening back pain, progressively poor urinary stream and urinary frequency. The serum PSA was 1000 ng/ml.

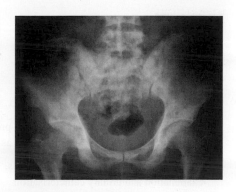

A. What abnormality can you observe in the X-ray?

B. What is the diagnosis?

C. What is PSA?

D. What other conditions may cause this elevation?

E. What options are there to manage the patient's back pain?

F. How may we manage his urinary problem?

Q9.14
This is an X-ray of a 66-year-old man who had developed gross haematuria.

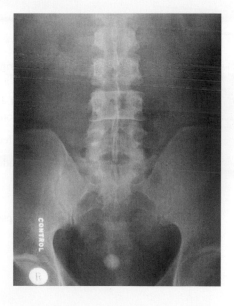

A. What abnormality can be seen in the X-ray?

B. What are the various aetiologies?

C. Who are most commonly affected?

D. What other symptoms is he likely to be have?

E. How may the condition be treated?

Answers

A9.13

A. Osteosclerotic bone deposits.

B. Stage 4 prostate cancer.

C. It is prostatic acid phosphotase and is produced by normal and malignant prostatic ductal and acinar epithelial cells. It acts as a tumour marker.

D. Benign prostatic hyperplasia, prostatis, post-urinary retention, post-digital rectal examination and urinary catheterisation.

E. Hormonal manipulation (deprivation of androgens/testosterone, androgen blockade with oestrogen diethylstilbestrol, LHRH agonists or surgical castration) and radiotherapy.

F. Transurethral resection of prostate (TURP).

A9.14

A. Bladder calculus.

B. **Primary**: develops in sterile urine (originates in the kidney and passes down the ureter to the bladder.

   Secondary: occurs in the presence of infection, bladder outflow obstruction, and impaired bladder emptying or foreign body.

C. Males are six times more likely to be affected.

D. Frequency, sensation of incomplete bladder emptying, pain (strangury), interruption of urinary stream and urinary infection.

E. 1. Treat the underlying cause.
   2. Litholapexy/Vesicolithotomy/lithotripsy.

Q9.15
This is an X-ray of a 60-year-old man.

A. What is the abnormality seen in the picture?

B. How useful are plain abdominal X-rays in diagnosing the condition?

C. How do you think he may have presented?

D. What are the possible complications of this condition?

E. What is the therapy for this condition?

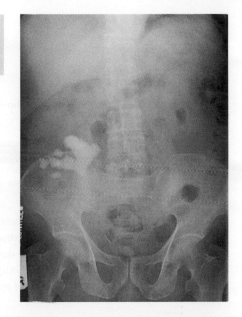

Q9.16
The 70-year-old man experienced pain and was unable to pass urine.

A. What is your finding, based on this picture?

B. How may the diagnosis be confirmed?

C. What are the possible causes?

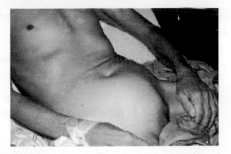

Answers

A9.15

A. Right renal calculi (staghorn).

B. Ninety percent of these stones are radio-opaque as they contain either calcium or cystine.

C. Stones in the renal pelvis may be asymptomatic or cause ureteric colic as they pass down the ureter. Haematuria may also occur.

D. Hydronephrosis, infection (pyonephrosis or pyelonephritis), haematuria and renal impairment.

E. Small stones have an 80% chance of being passed out. Larger stones like this one warrant intervention. Options include extracorporeal shock-wave lithotripsy (ESWL) in which shock energy is used to break down the stone. If ESWL fails or the stones are too large, percutaneous nephrolithotripsy (PCNL) can be considered. If these options fails, open surgery in the form of pyelolithotomy may be performed.

A9.16

A. A large mass in the lower abdomen.

A full bladder from urinary retention, which will be dull to percussion and tender to palpation, needs to be excluded before any further investigations is carried out.

B. A trans-abdominal ultrasound can confirm a full bladder. Catheterisation of the patient, either per-urethral or suprapubic yielding a high urine volume will be confirmation.

C. Bladder outflow obstruction (stone or clot), urethral stricture, urethritis, phimosis, neurogenic, faecal impaction, post-operative pain or drugs (antihistamine, anticholinergic, tricyclic anti-depressants).

Q9.17
The 60-year-old man had surgery for bladder cancer.

A. What are the contents of the bag?

B. What kind of surgery did the patient undergo?

C. What are the potential complications of this procedure?

D. What other modes of diversion are there?

E. What are the metabolic consequences of this form of diversion?

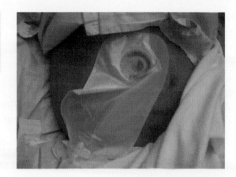

Q9.18
A 43-year-old man was investigated for recurrent urinary tract infections.

A. What abnormality can be seen in these scans?

B. What factors could have led to the abnormality?

C. Which other imaging procedures may be performed?

D. What symptoms might the patient have?

E. What are the indications for surgical intervention?

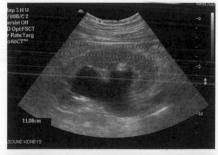

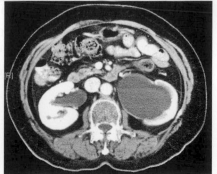

Answers

A9.17

A. Urine.

B. Radical cystectomy with permanent urinary external diversion – ileal conduit. The ureters are implanted into a short segment of ileum or less commonly, the colon.

C. Ureteroileal stricture, which may be prevented by spatulation of the distal ureters.

D. Internal: ureterosigmoidostomy, bladder reconstruction with lengths of various bowel or bladder augmentation.

E. The biochemical changes are due to the resorption of solutes (chloride and urea) in the small bowel and diminishing tubular function due to recurrent pyelonephritis from ascending infection. The severity depends on area of bowel and length of time exposed to urine. Typically, hyperchloraemic acidosis with potassium depletion occurs.

A9.18

A. Bilateral hydronephrosis.

B. It is often a pathology that causes bladder outflow obstruction and thus bilateral hydronephrosis. Causes include retroperitoneal tumours (lymphoma or sarcoma) or fibrosis, pelvic tumours, and extensive bladder tumours or larger bladder stones.

C. Renal scanning with Technetium-labeled dimercaptosuccinic acid (DMSA) allows assessment of renal function.

Technetium-labeled diethylenetriminepentaacetic acid (DTPA) scans can provide information on renal perfusion, function and presence of obstruction.

D. They are mostly asymptomatic, except for a dull ache. The kidneys are unlikely to be palpable because renal failure sets in before the kidneys become sufficiently large.

E. Recurrent bouts of renal pain, increasing hydronephrosis, evidence of parenchymal damage and infection.

Q9.19
The 30-year-old man presented with haematuria.

A. What pathology can be seen, based on picture A? What procedure was attempted?

B. What are its possible causes?

C. What is the normal anatomical course of the structure?

D. What symptoms would the patient present?

E. What can be seen in picture B?

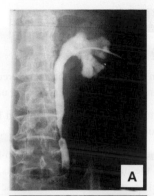

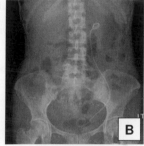

Answer

A9.19

A. An enlarged left ureter. A percutaneous nephrostomy (PCN) with an attempt to cannulate beyond the narrowing under radiological guidance.

B. Causes of unilateral obstruction include luminal (sloughed papilla, stone or clots), mural (tumour and stricture) and extrinsic (retroperitoneal fibrosis).

C. The ureter passes over the genito-femoral nerve and under the gonadal vessels, lateral to the inferior mesenteric vessels, deep to the left colic vessels, crosses the brim of pelvis, runs over the external iliac vessels and under the vas dererens (in males), turns medially at the level of the ischial spine and enters the bladder inferiolaterally.

D. Acute obstruction can present with pain but chronic obstruction may produce vague symptoms.

E. A double-J ureteric stent in position across the narrowing.

Chapter 10

PLASTIC AND RECONSTRUCTIVE SURGERY

Q10.1
This 67-year-old male had a slow-growing lesion over the left lower eyelid for the past 10 years.

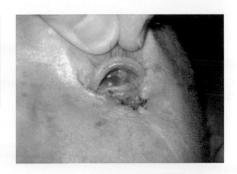

A. Describe the clinical features.

B. What factors would you consider when diagnosing the patient?

C. What aetiological factors may predispose one to developing this lesion?

D. What are the various ways in which the lesion may present?

Q10.2
The baby was born with a birth mark, as seen in picture A. Picture B shows the result after treatment.

A. What is the birthmark called?

B. What is the common anatomical distribution of these lesions?

C. What is the dermatome distribution in this patient?

D. Is there any intracranial association?

E. What association is there with varicose veins?

F. How can we manage the lesion?

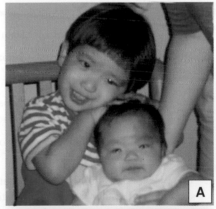

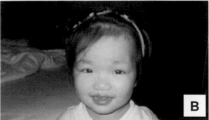

Answers

A10.1

A. There is a large ulcer destroying the lower eyelid and invading the sclera/globe of the left eye.

B. Basal cell carcinoma (BCC).

C.   i. UV induced mutation of p53 gene and tumour suppressor genes,
    ii. Arsenic exposure,
    iii. Immunosuppression.

D. The commonest subtype is nodular BCC. Other clinical variants of BCC include: superficial BCC, pigmented BCC, cystic BCC, micronodular BCC, morpheaform/sclerosing BCC.

A10.2

A. Capillary haemangioma (Port wine stain).

B. They often conform to the sensory dermatomes, especially when on the face.

C. 5th cranial nerve-ophthalmic division.

D. Sturge-Weber Syndrome is described when there is ipsilateral meningeal involvement in conjunction with hemifacial hemangiomas.

E. Klippel-Trenaunay Syndrome consists of a triad of limb hypertrophy, varicose veins and port wine staining.

F. These skin lesions do not regress spontaneously but surface lasers have been used, showing good results (as seen in this patient in picture B).

Q10.3
This is a 30-year-old man with a lump over the lip.

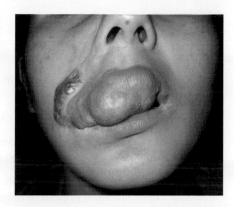

A. Describe the lesion.

B. What is your diagnosis?

C. What is the natural history of this lesion?

D. What problems will develop if the lesion grows bigger?

Q10.4
These are lesions found on two different patients.

A. Describe the lesions.

B. What would you look out for when carrying out a medical examination?

C. What is the most likely diagnosis?

D. What are the possible differential diagnoses?

E. How should the conditions be treated?

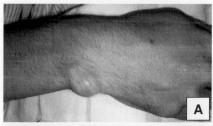

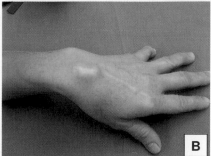

Answers

A10.3

A. There is a large erythematous lesion with visible venous channels in the background of an enlarged of upper lip.

B. Cavernous arteriovenous malformation (AVM).

C. The onset is usually after birth. The development is divided into proliferative (rapid growth for 3–9 months, up to 18 months) and involutive phase (over 2–6 years).

D. Large lesions may be associated with ptosis, obstruction of vision, high-output cardiac failure, thrombocytopenia or hemolytic anaemia and frank bleeding.

A10.4

A. Both are hemispherical lesions, at 2 x 2 cm over the ulnar aspect (picture A) and the dorsum of the wrist (picture B). There is no overlying skin change.

B. Test for its consistency; transillumination; its mobility with respect to tendons; slip sign; and whether it occurs in other areas or is confined to the region of the wrist.

C. Ganglion. It is a synovial-fluid filled cyst arising from synovial tissue in relation to joints or tendons and is often in the dorsal aspect. It occurs at any age but is uncommon in children. They are usually painless, firm, and asymptomatic and develop around the wrist.

D. A lipoma, epidermal cyst or bursa.

E. One third rule – a third gets smaller, a third remains the same and the other third enlarges. Occasionally, a blow to it causes it to disappear but up to 50% of them recur.

Q10.5
This lesion was found on the thigh of a 30-year-old lady.

A. Describe this lesion.

B. How are pigmented lesions classified histologically?

C. What is the most likely diagnosis?

D. What causes the pigmentation?

E. What is the recommended treatment of the lesion?

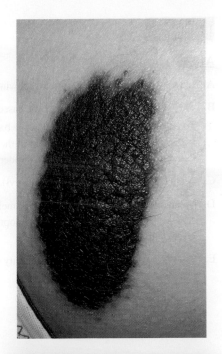

Q10.6
This picture shows the forehead and hairline of a 70-year-old patient.

A. Describe the abnormal findings.

B. What is the diagnosis?

C. What is its natural history?

D. What can be seen histologically?

E. How can these lesions be managed?

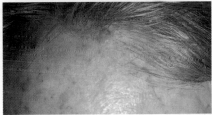

Answers

A10.5

A. Large pigmented lesion with hair growing from the substance.

B. They are divided into three groups, based on the position of the melanocytes.
   Junctional: proliferation is within the basal layer.
   Intradermal: proliferation is deep to the basal layer within the dermis.
   Compound: both junctional and intradermal.

C. Giant Hairy Naevus. (intradermal naevi).

D. Melanin is the pigment produced by melanocytes, which are derived from the neural crest cells that migrate during development and are scattered throughout the basal layer of the skin epidermis.

E. Complete excision due to the possibility of malignant change over time.

A10.6

A. There are multiple macular/papular hyperkeratotic spots over the forehead with pigmentation.

B. Solar keratosis.

C. It is a pre-malignant condition.

D. Areas of hyperkeratosis. They undergo malignant change when there is cellular dysplasia involving the full thickness of epithelium.

E. Laser vapourisation and regular follow-up surveillance, reduced sun exposure and regular use of sun blocks prevents its development.

Q10.7
This lesion has been present since birth. There is no history of bleeding, but occasional oozing of straw-coloured fluid.

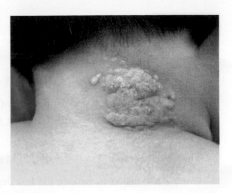

A. What abnormality can be seen?

B. What is the most likely diagnosis?

C. What is the natural history?

D. How can we manage the patient?

Q10.8
The 58-year-old male had a lesion that grew for the past 3 years. He suffered burns on his face 20 years ago.

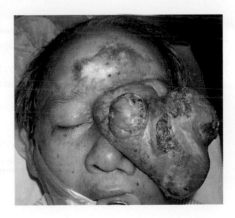

A. What is the most likely diagnosis and how would you confirm it?

B. Why did the lesion develop on the patient's face?

C. What problems may this lesion cause?

D. If the lesion is confined to the face, how would you manage the condition?

Answers

A10.7

A. Multiple pinkish raised lesions over back of neck.

B. Lymphangioma. They are collections of lymphatic tissue with variable amount of fibrosis and lymphocytic infiltration. It can be solid or cutaneous. This lesion is a mixture.

C. They tend to increase in size as the child grows and show little regression.

D. Complete excision to include the full depth of skin to avoid recurrence. If lesion is too large, sclerosants may be used initially to induce involution.

A10.8

A. Squamous cell carcinoma. Incisional biopsy.

B. Marjolin transformation of burn scar. Typically, the longer the duration of the chronic irritated scar, the more likely the transformation.

C. Obstruction/invasion into left eye, blockage of upper airway on left side and invasion into cranium.

D. Radical excision (with reconstruction) and radiotherapy. Chemotherapy can be considered. After treatment, regular follow-up is required.

Q10.9
The 74-year-old woman had multiple skin lesions for many years.

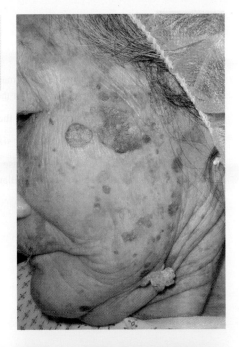

A. Describe the lesions on her face.

B. What would be your main concern regarding the lesion at her jaw line?

C. What symptoms or signs may point to sinister change?

D. How would you manage the lesion at her jaw line?

Q10.10
This is a scalp lesion on a 16-year-old.

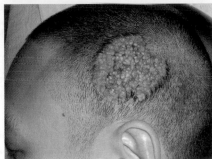

A. Describe this lesion.

B. What is the diagnosis?

C. How did this lesion develop?

D. What would you expect to find upon histological examination of the lesion?

Answers

A10.9

A. Seborrhoeic keratosis over the zygomatic prominence, solar keratosis over the forehead, cheek and a cutaneous horn at the left jaw line.

B. Squamous cell carcinoma at the base of the cutaneous horn.

C. Tenderness at base and lesions of larger size.

D. Excision of the lesion, including the base and adequate margins, evaluate for distant metastases and regular follow-up surveillance.

A10.10

A. Well-circumscribed salmon – brown coloured lesion with a bosselated appearance.

B. Sebaceous naevus of Jadassohn.

C. The growth is related to hormonal fluctuations – it has a raised appearance at birth, flattens during childhood and rises again during puberty. Up to 5–7% of cases may develop into basal cell carcinoma.

D. Papillomatous hyperplasia present in the epidermis with numerous sebaceous glands in the dermis. Apocrine glands, small hair follicles and buds of basaloid cells will also be present.

Q10.11
This man had a lesion on the sole of his right foot for 2 years. It recently ulcerated and he also discovered a lump in his right groin.

A. Describe the lesion on the foot.

B. What is the diagnosis?

C. Where did the condition originate from?

D. How would you stage the lesion? What staging classification would you use?

E. What are the other prognostic factors?

F. Which principle risk factors are responsible?

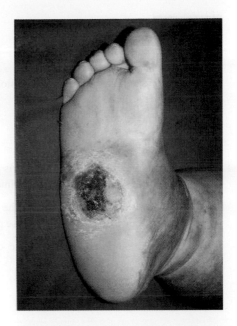

Q10.12
This is a 30-year-old man who presented with a lump over the back that had increased in size over 1 month.

A. Describe the lesion?

B. What is the most likely diagnosis?

C. Which symptoms and signs are sinister?

D. What pathological types are they classified as and which are most common?

E. How do we manage them?

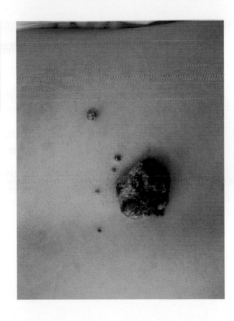

Answers

A10.11

A. Irregular hyper-pigmented ulcerated lesion over the right sole, 3 x 4 cm in size with surrounding infiltration.

B. Malignant melanoma.

C. Melanocytes.

D. Systemic staging is by CT thorax, pelvis & abdomen. Local staging is by Breslow's tumour thickness. The thickness in millimetres is used to predict outcome.

E. Ulceration, male gender, lesions over the trunk compared to extremities and middle-aged patients are associated with a worse prognosis.

F. UV light exposure and previous large congenital melanocytic naevi, which have transformed.

A10.12

A. There is a 5 x 5 cm nodular lesion with multiple surrounding satellite nodules.

B. Malignant melanoma.

C. Itchiness, bleeding, increasing pigmentation, ulceration and development of satellite nodules.

D. The two most common are the superficial spreading and nodular. The others are lentigo maligna melanoma and acral lentigenous melanoma.

E. Surgical excision with adequate margins of 2–3cm is the mainstay of treatment. Other forms of treatment include immunotherapy, chemotherapy (systemic and local perfusion) and radiotherapy.

Q10.13
This is a 35-year-old female with a growing mass on the left side of her face.

A. What problems is she likely to encounter?

B. What is your diagnosis?

C. Define the condition.

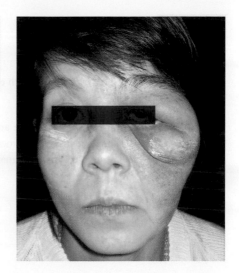

Q10.14

A. What is seen on this patient in picture A and what is the diagnosis?

B. What is its genetic disposition?

C. Are these lesions potentially malignant?

D. What other tumours are associated with this condition?

E. What can be seen on the neck of this patient in picture B and what is its association with this disease?

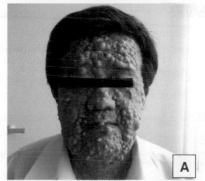

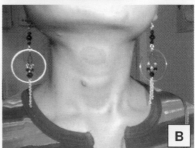

Answers

A10.13

A. Left visual disturbance, interference with chewing, left face distortion.

B. Plexiform Neurofibromatosis.

C. It is a primary abnormality in which an area of the body is involved in a diffuse and often extensive subcutaneous enlargement. The overlying skin is thickened and pigmented. It may resemble lymphoedema.

A10.14

A. There are multiple neurofibromas over his face. The diagnosis is type 1 neurofibromatosis – Von Recklinghausen's Disease.

B. Autosomal dominant trait.

C. 5% of them develop neurofibrosarcoma.

D. Ganglioneuromas, phaeochromocytomas, gliomas and meningiomas.

E. Café-au-lait spots. They are characteristic and diagnostic of Von Recklinghausen's Disease if there are more than six or a patch of more than 1.5 cm across.

Q10.15
The 46-year-old lady had a lesion over the nose.

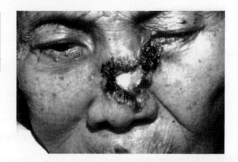

A. What abnormality can you observe?

B. What is the diagnosis?

C. Where did it develop from?

D. Who are most at risk?

E. What will be the natural history if the lesion is left untreated?

Q10.16
This is a 70-year-old lady with a nose lesion.

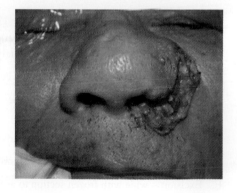

A. Describe the features of the lesion on this patient.

B. What is the diagnosis? Provide differential diagnoses.

C. What are the predisposing factors?

D. What are precursors of this disease?

E. How should the patient be managed?

Answers

A10.15

A. There is a pigmented ulcerated lesion over the nose, extending to the left lower eyelid, 2 x 4 cm in size, irregular margins with rolled edges (rodent ulcer).

B. Pigmented basal cell carcinoma.

C. Malignant change in the basal layer of the epidermis.

D. Males are twice more likely to be affected as well as those who have had ultraviolet light exposure.

E. They are locally malignant and undergo steady, slow and destructive enlargement. For this patient, there would be invasion of the left eye globe and into the intra-cranial cavity via the orbit. They generally do not metastasise.

A10.16

A. Large ulcer at left nostril with everted edges, 2 x 3 cm, irregular margins, slough in the base and the left alar almost completely destroyed.

B. Squamous cell carcinoma (SCC); Basal cell carcinoma, and Charga's Disease.

   SCC arise from the keratinocytes in the epidermis and grow rapidly with anaplasia, local invasion and metastases.

C. Exposure to sunlight, chemical hydrocarbons, arsenic and chrome compounds.

D. Bowen's Disease (squamous cell carcinoma in situ) and solar keratosis.

E. Excision – wide with frozen section to ascertain clearance; radiotherapy.

Q10.17
The 30-year-old lady had been trapped in a burning room.

A. What is seen in picture A?

B. What would be your concerns during the initial resuscitation?

C. What are the guidelines to fluid resuscitation?

D. Despite endotracheal intubation, why is there difficulty in ventilation of the patient?

E. What procedure was performed in picture B?

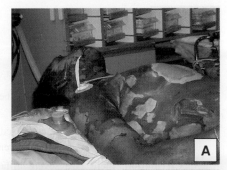

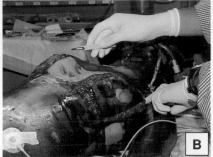

Q10.18
These are intra-operative pictures.

A. What surgeries did these patients undergo?

B. Define these procedures.

C. What types of surgery are there to treat these conditions and what are their advantages and disadvantages?

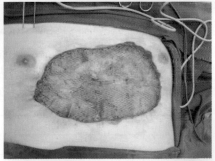

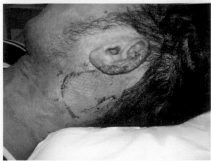

Answers

A10.17

A. There are extensive burns on this patient.

B. **1: Airway**: a burned airway can become swollen and cause upper airway obstruction.

    2: Breathing: Inhalation injuries caused by minute particles within the thick smoke that are carried down to the lung parenchyma.

    3: Circulation: there is a severe inflammatory reaction with increased vascular permeability.

C. Area and thickness of burned area, and the time following the burn insult.

D. She had suffered full-thickness circumferential burns of her chest wall, which impeded chest expansion.

E. An escharotomy.

A10.18

A. Skin grafting. They had STSG as seen by the mesh-like appearance.

B. Total detachment of tissue from one part of the body and transferred to another part where it must establish its own blood supply.

C. Split-thickness skin graft (STSG) and full-thickness graft (FTSG).

	STSG	FTSG
Take	Reliable	Needs a well-vascularised clean bed
Adnexal structures	Absent	Preserved
Donor site	Less area needed due to meshing and allowed to re-epithelised	Meshing is difficult and wounds are closed primarily
Recipient site	Hyperpigmentation and shrinkage	Less likely to shrink

Q10.19
An 8-year-old developed an upper lip lump after minor trauma.

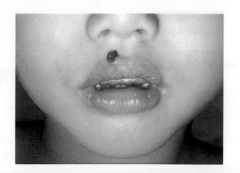

A. Describe this lesion.

B. What is the diagnosis?

C. What is the definition?

D. What would you recommend for the treatment of the lesion?

Q10.20
This lady complained of a lump over her earlobe.

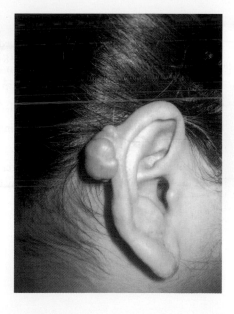

A. What are the stages of wound healing?

B. What is the definition of a hypertrophic scar?

C. What can be seen in the picture?

D. What is its definition?

E. How may we manage this condition?

Answers

A10.19

A. There is a small reddish lump of granulation tissue, 2 x 2 mm in size over the upper lip with contact bleeding.

B. Pyogenic granuloma.

C. It is an exuberant growth of granulation tissue due to abnormal inflammatory response, which resulted in the polypoid lesion.

D. Resolution is slow and excision is often recommended.

A10.20

A. There are four stages: coagulation (immediate), inflammation (1–4 days), fibroplasia (up to 3 weeks) and remodelling (up to 18 months).

B. Excessive build-up of scar tissue confined to the initial boundary of the wound.

C. Keloid formation over the right ear lobe.

D. Excessive build-up of scar tissue that invades the normal skin beyond the original boundary of the wound.

E. Treatment is difficult. Options include repeated local steroid injections after excision of the lesion. Low dose radiotherapy may be attempted.

Chapter 11

ENDOCRINE SURGERY

Q11.1
This 40-year-old man underwent a CT scan to investigate a vague abdominal pain.

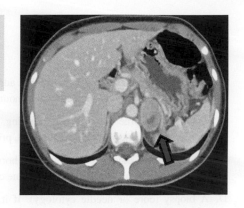

A. The scan shows a mass. What is it? What would you call this clinical condition?

B. What are the possible diagnoses?

C. What initial investigations are appropriate?

D. What kind of investigation should not be performed?

Q11.2
This 40-year-old lady had a total thyroidectomy.

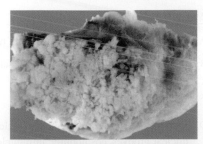

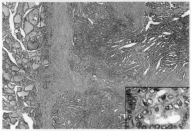

A. What can be seen from the gross specimen?

B. What can be seen microscopically?

C. What is the diagnosis?

D. What are the other microscopic features of this tumour?

E. What are some histologic variants?

F. Who are more at risk, how does this condition spread and what is a known risk factor?

Answers

A11.1

A. There is a tumour arising from the left adrenal gland. It is an adrenal incidentaloma (the incidental finding of an adrenal tumour).

B. Conn's Syndrome (aldosterone-secreting tumour), Cushing's Syndrome (cortisol-secreting tumour), phaeochromocytoma, primary adrenal cancer and metastasis.

C. Evaluation for evidence of abnormal hormonal hypersecretion – serum renin and aldosterone, serum cortisol, 24-hour urine catecholamines.

D. A biopsy (core or needle cytology). If it were a malignant lesion, it could cause seeding to the tumour and if it were a phaeochromocytoma, a hypertensive crisis could be precipitated.

    Occasionally a biopsy may be indicated to confirm adrenal metastasis.

A11.2

A. The left side of the specimen shows a tumour with a papillary architecture.

B. Infiltrative papillary tumour with sclerotic stroma. The high power inset shows nuclear crowding and clearing.

C. Papillary thyroid cancer.

D. Evidence of hypochromic empty nuclei devoid of nucleoli (Orphan Annie eyes) and nuclear grooves, eosinophilic intranuclear inclusions and psammoma bodies.

E. Encapsulated variant, follicular variant and tall cell (tall cell subtypes are associated with a poorer prognosis).

F. Women between 20–40 years of age. They have a propensity for lymphatic invasion. Ionising radiation is a known risk factor.

Q11.3
This 35-year-old man underwent investigation for hypertension. He was found to be hypokalaemic.

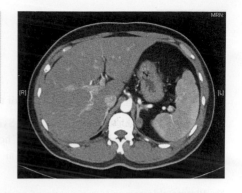

A. What initial investigation would you carry out?

B. What does the CT scan show?

C. What is the diagnosis?

D. What is the confirming biochemical test?

E. What is the pre-operative treatment?

Q11.4
This is a specimen from a 40-year-old lady who underwent an adrenalectomy for hypertension.

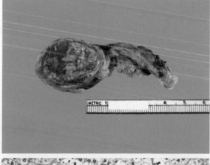

A. What can be observed about the gross specimen?

B. What can be observed about the microscopic specimen?

C. What is the most likely diagnosis?

D. What would suggest that the lesion is a carcinoma?

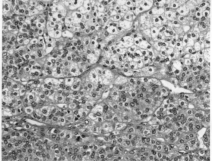

Answers

A11.3

A. Serum aldosterone (not a CT scan).

B. A tumour arising from the medial limb of the left adrenal gland.

C. Primary hyperaldosteronism. (Conn's Syndrome). It is characterised by the over-production of the mineralocorticoid hormone aldosterone. Aldosterone causes increase in sodium and water retention and potassium excretion in the kidneys, resulting in hypertension.

D. Plasma aldosterone to renin ratio of greater than 30. Measuring aldosterone alone is not adequate to diagnose Conn's Syndrome.

E. Spironolactone (anti-aldosterone diuretic).

A11.4

A. A solitary lesion arising from the adrenal gland. The cut surface is bright yellow, reflecting high lipid content.

B. Trabeculae of cells with clear-foamy to granular cytoplasm, separated by thin fibrovascular septa.

C. Adrenal cortical adenoma.

D. Hallmarks of carcinoma are its large size, evidence of local invasion, poor differentiation to anaplastic cells, vascular invasion and lymphatic spread.

Q11.5
This 50-year-old lady had a total thyroidectomy for a follicular thyroid carcinoma.

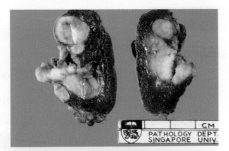

A. What can be observed about the gross specimen?

B. What features suggest malignancy?

C. In which way does this condition most commonly spread?

D. How useful is pre-operative fine needle cytological examination of the lesion?

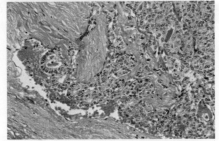

Q11.6
This 19-year-old girl presented with repeated episodes of palpitations, headache and episodic diaphoresis.

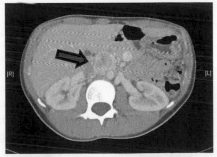

A. What can be seen from the scan?

B. What is the diagnosis?

C. What are the associated risk factors?

D. What biochemical abnormalities might she have?

E. What is essential during the pre-operative preparation?

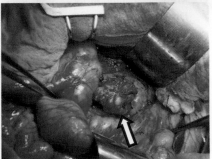

Answers

A11.5

A. Infiltrative pale nodules within the thyroid gland.

B. Evidence of capsular and vascular invasion on histology.

C. Haematogenous spread to bone, lung and liver.

D. Cytological examination to distinguish follicular carcinoma from an adenoma is very unreliable. Papillary carcinoma may be diagnosed with identification of characteristic nuclear features.

A11.6

A. A well-circumscribed heterogenous lesion sitting between the aorta and inferior vena cava.

B. Phaeochromocytoma. Tumour of the adrenal medulla and sympathetic ganglion (chromoffin cell lines) that produce catecholamines. This patient had an extra-adrenal phaeochromocytoma (extra-adrenal paraganglioma). These tumours are traditionally known as "10%" tumours; the percentage of which are bilateral, malignant, extra-adrenal, arising in childhood, familial and recurrence after excision.

C. MEN 2, family history, Von Recklinghausen Disease and Von Hippel-Lindau Disease.

D. Elevated urine Vanillylmandelic acid (VMA), metanephrine and non-metanephrine.

E. Increase intravascular volume with adequate alpha-blockade.

Q11.7
This is a 52-year-old man who presented with hypercalcaemia.

A. What are the common causes of hypercalcaemia?

B. What symptoms might he have?

C. Which pre-operative blood test may have pre-empted the radiological investigation?

D. What radiological investigation was carried in picture A and what does it show?

E. What is the diagnosis, based on picture B?

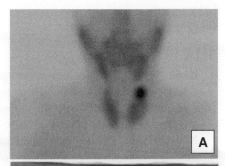

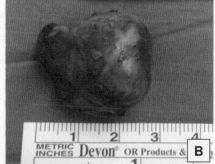

Q11.8
The lady had recurrent hyperparathyroidism after a four-gland parathyroidectomy.

A. What is the embryologic origin of the parathyroid glands?

B. How is refractory renal hyperparathyrodism managed?

C. Apart from their usual position posterior to the thyroid gland, where else are they situated?

D. What can be seen in the sestamibi and CT scans?

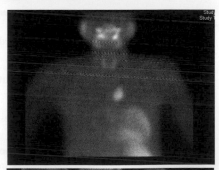

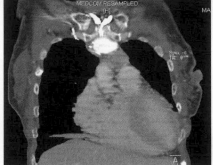

Answers

A11.7

A. **Endocrine** – Hyperparathyrodism (primary and renal), hyperthyroidism and Addison's Disease. **Malignancy** – bone metastasis, haematological (myeloma, leukaemia and lymphoma), solid tumours (lung carcinoma) and paraneoplastic syndromes. **Increase intake** – milk-alkali syndrome, vitamin D intoxication. **Miscellaneous** – granulomatous diseases (sarcoidosis, tuberculosis), lithium and thiazide use, familial hypocalciuric hypercalcaemia (FHH).

B. "Bones, stones, groans, and moans (psychiatric overtones)."

C. An elevated serum parathyroid hormone (PTH).

D. The Sestamibi parathyroid function scan shows a hyperfunctioning superior left parathyroid gland.

E. Primary hyperparathyroidism secondary to a parathyroid tumour (adenoma is more common than carcinoma). A normal parathyroid gland is 0.5 to 1 cm.

A11.8

A. Superior and inferior glands are derived from the 4th pharyngeal and 3rd pharyngeal pouch respectively.

B. Total parathyroidectomy and re-implantation or subtotal parathyroidectomy if the patients anticipate a renal transplant.

C. Based on their embryological descent, their positions can vary. Other positions include within the thyroid gland, thymus/mediastinum, carotid sheath, tracheoesophageal groove and retro-oesophagus.

D. A hyperfunctioning parathyroid gland in the mediastinum.

Q11.9
The 32-year-old man had a neck lump.

A. How would you know if this is a goitre, based on picture A?

B. How can we distinguish it from a thyroglossal cyst?

C. Where is the embryological origin of the thyroid?

D. What problems can develop if the lesion is left alone?

E. What treatment would you recommend?

F. What has been performed prior to surgery in picture B?

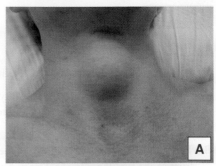

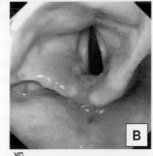

VC

Q11.10
This 55-year-old lady had frequent fainting spells which were relieved by eating.

A. What symptoms was she describing?

B. Which blood investigations would you have performed?

C. What did the localising CT show?

D. How common is this condition?

E. What is this condition often associated with?

F. What is the treatment?

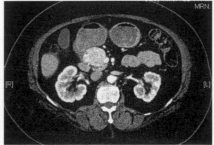

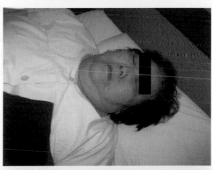

Answers

A11.9

A. The thyroid moves with swallowing as it is attached to the larynx.

B. Ask him to stick out his tongue. A thyroglossal cyst would move with swallowing and move up with protrusion of the tongue. A thyroid would not move with the protrusion of the tongue.

C. The thyroid descends caudally from the foramen caecum and reaches its position in front of the first three tracheal rings by week 7 of gestation. Persistence of this duct gives rise to a cystic mass (thyroglossal cyst).

D. It may enlarge or get infected.

E. Sistrunk procedure. It involves resection of the mass, a central portion of the hyoid bone and a small block of the tongue base.

F. Pre-operative evaluation of vocal cord function is necessary because there is a possibility of inadvertent recurrent laryngeal nerve injury during surgery.

A11.10

A. Whipple's triad. Hypoglycaemic symptoms produced by fasting, proven hypogylcaemia and relief of symptoms by administration of glucose (note that her obesity can be explained by her increased food intake).

B. Glucose and insulin levels during fast (fasting hypoglycaemia with inappropriately high levels of insulin – 72-hour fast).

C. Insulinoma in the head of pancreas. It is a tumour of the pancreas arising from the beta cells which, while retaining the ability to synthesise and secrete insulin, is autonomous of the normal feedback mechanism.

D. It is uncommon (one in 100,000).

E. Multiple Endocrine Neoplasia (MEN) 1 Syndrome (pituitary, pancreas and parathyroid).

F. Diazoxide to suppress insulin release, followed by surgical resection.

Q11.11
This 30-year-old lady experienced discomfort in the neck.

A. Describe what you see in picture A.

B. What are the differential diagnoses?

C. What examination would you perform next?

D. What investigation would you perform if a thyroid lump is confirmed?

E. What are the differential diagnoses of a thyroid nodule?

F. What procedure had been performed for the patient, according to picture B?

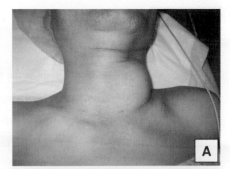

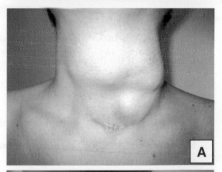

Q11.12
This patient had a previous total thyroidectomy for thyroid cancer.

A. What can be seen in this picture A?

B. What is the most likely diagnosis?

C. He presented with hoarseness of voice. What are the causes?

D. What can we do to confirm the diagnosis?

E. What has been performed for the patient, as seen in picture B?

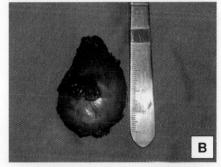

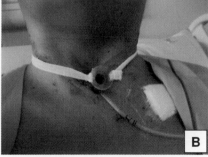

Answers

A11.11

A. A mass in the left anterior triangle of the neck.

B. Thyroid nodule, lymphadenopathy, thyroglossal cyst, lipoma.

C. Ask the patient to swallow. A thyroid lump would move with swallowing.

D. An ultrasound can obtain further characteristics of this lesion, thyroid function test to rule out a toxic nodule and fine needle aspiration and cytological examination.

E. **Benign**: cyst, adenoma, thyroiditis.
    Malignant: carcinoma, lymphoma.

F. Thyroid lobectomy.

A11.12

A. Multiple lumps/masses in the anterior neck and a previous surgical scar.

B. Recurrence of the thyroid cancer.

C. Involvement of the tumour with the recurrent laryngeal nerve or direct invasion into the larynx.

D. Laryngoscopy to visualise the vocal cords and the integrity of the larynx.

E. Resection of the recurrence and a total laryngectomy (note the presence of the trachostomy and enteral feeding tube).

Q11.13
This is a 60-year-old lady who presented with a long-standing neck lump.

A. What symptoms could she be complaining of?

B. What clinical manoeuvre would you perform?

C. What investigation would you carry out prior to surgery?

D. What can be seen in the chest X-ray?

E. What potential complications might develop after surgery?

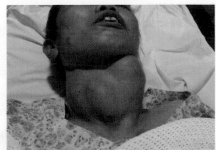

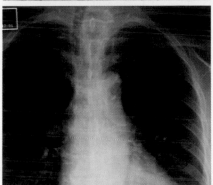

Q11.14
This 80-year-old lady had a lump in her neck that moved when she swallowed.

A. What can be seen in the pictures?

B. What is the diagnosis?

C. What are the different histology subtypes?

D. How can we manage the patient?

E. What is the post-operative adjuvant treatment?

F. How can we monitor for recurrent disease?

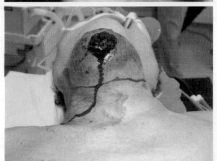

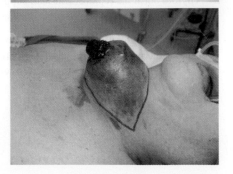

Answers

A11.13

A. Respiratory obstruction, hoarseness (vocal cord palsy) and syncope.

B. Elicit Pemberton's sign where elevation of the patient's arms may lead to venous congestion and stridor if there is retrosternal extension of the goitre.

C. Thyroid function test, CXR and CT of the neck.

D. Tracheal deviation.

E. Haemorrhage and tracheomalacia (from long-standing obstruction) giving rise to upper airway compromise, injury to the recurrent laryngeal nerve and external branch of superior laryngeal nerve and injury to parathyroid glands.

A11.14

A. A mass arising from the central portion of her neck that has ulcerated through the skin and caused bleeding.

B. Thyroid carcinoma.

C. Papillary (70%), Follicular (20%), Medullary (5%), Hurthle (4%) and anaplastic (1%).

D. Total thyroidectomy and neck dissection if there are palpable lymphadenopathies.

E. Thyroid hormone replacement with suppression of TSH, and post-operative low dose radio-Iodine131 to locate residual disease and high dose to ablate them.

F. Serum thyroglobulin is a protein within the thyroid follicle. After a total thyroidectomy, the thyroglobulin levels will be unmeasurable. Any elevation of serum thyroglobulin levels during follow-up would indicate a recurrence.

Q11.15
This 23-year-old lady is hyperthyroid and has a prominent left thyroid nodule.

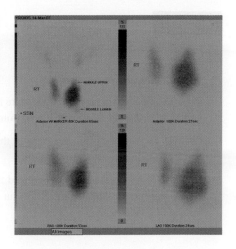

A. What investigation was performed, based on the picture?

B. Why was it performed?

C. How can this patient be managed?

D. If this patient underwent surgery, what factors do we have to take into consideration and how can we optimise the results?

Q11.16
This 35-year-old man presented with a diffuse thyroid swelling.

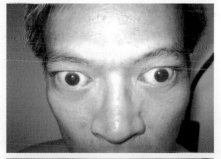

A. What is the diagnosis?

B. What is the definition of this condition?

C. What is its epidemiology?

D. What are the eye signs he might have?

E. How is diagnosis made?

F. What are the modes of management?

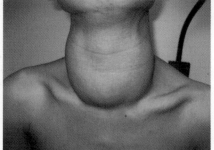

Answers

A11.15

A. Radio-Iodine131 uptake scan.

B. To ascertain whether her thyrotoxic state is due to the dominant nodule or if she has a global hyperthyroid gland with a cold dominant nodule.

C. Options include surgical removal of the toxic nodule (left lobectomy), medical control or radioactive iodine ablation.

D. We have to render the patient euthyroid to prevent the triggering of a thyroid storm, which may be life-threatening. This can be assisted with beta-adrenergic blockade, thioamides and iodine.

A11.16

A. Graves' Disease.

B. Excessive circulating auto-antibodies that stimulate thyroid-stimulating hormone (TSH) receptors on follicular cells of the thyroid. It is characterised by a diffuse goitre and hyperthyroidism.

C. Females are 6 times more commonly affected. It occurs most during the 3rd to 5th decade of one's life. There is also a family preponderance.

D. Exophthalmos, lower eyelid retraction, lid lag (stimulation of the levator palpebrae superiores), chemosis and pre-orbital oedema.

E. Increased T3, T4 and decreased TSH, 90% will have raised anti-TSH receptor antibodies and 70% will have raised thyroid peroxidase (TPO) antibodies.

F. Medical blockade, radioiodine and surgical resection. Each mode has its advantages and disadvantages and should be tailored to the patient's needs and preferences.

Chapter 12

PAEDIATRIC SURGERY

K Prabhakaran

Dale L S K Loh

Q12.1
The 6-week-old male infant presented with non-bilious projectile vomiting. A visible swelling can be seen on the body, moving from left to right.

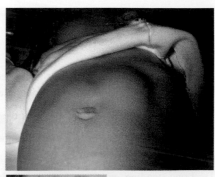

A. What is the diagnosis and what is the definition?

B. What radiological investigation has been done and what does it reveal?

C. What other imaging procedures can be done to confirm the diagnosis?

D. What biochemical abnormality is commonly associated with this condition?

E. How can we mange this condition?

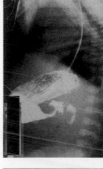
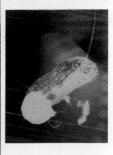

Q12.2
This 1-year-old boy was born prematurely.

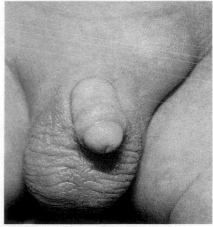

A. What abnormality can be seen?

B. What is the diagnosis?

C. How common is the condition and who are usually affected?

D. What are the possible differential diagnoses?

E. How would this condition be managed?

Answers

A12.1

A. Congenital pyloric stenosis. It is defined as an idiopathic thickening and elongation of the pylorus that produces gastric outlet obstruction.

B. Barium meal. It shows narrowing of the pylorus.

C. An ultrasound can be performed to look for the pyloric diameter, wall width and pyloric channel length.

D. Long-standing vomiting will result in hypokalaemic hypochloraemia metabolic alkalosis due to loss of gastric acid, leading to dehydration and electrolyte imbalance.

E. Fredet-Ramstedt pyloromyotomy.

A12.2

A. A swelling in the left groin.

B. A left inguinal hernia. Inguinal hernias are the most common condition requiring surgery in childhood.

C. They are up to 8 times more common in boys and incidence is one in 50 live births. It is more common in premature babies.

D. Encysted hydrocoele of the cord, femoral hernia or undescended testis.

E. **Reducible** – elective repair with high ligation of sac through a low abdominal incision.

   Incarcerated – most can be reduced with gentle direct pressure on the hernia followed by elective surgery.

   Strangulated – emergent surgery is indicated.

Q12.3
This is an X-ray of a new-born baby who is "mucussy."

A. What is the most obvious abnormality in the X-ray?

B. What other investigation can help confirm the diagnosis?

C. What is the diagnosis and what other anomalies are associated with the condition?

D. What is the initial treatment?

E. What is the definitive treatment?

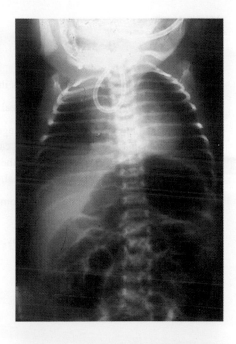

Q12.4
The 3-year-old infant presented with an abdominal mass and haematuria.

A. What are the three most common causes of abdominal masses in infants?

B. What is the diagnosis of this infant's condition?

C. Which features help distinguish this infant's tumour from other kinds of tumours?

D. What are the management options of this patient?

E. What are the best indicators of survival?

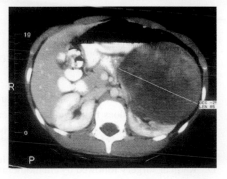

Answers

A12.3

A. A tube coiled in the oesophagus and gas in the intestines.

B. "Pouchogram" (contrast in the esophageal pouch).

C. Oesophageal atresia. A tracheo-oesophageal fistula occurs in more than 90%. Other birth defects may co-exist, commonly cardiac and occasionally in the anus, spinal column or kidneys. This is known as the VACTERL Syndrome (Vertebral column, Anorectal, Cardiac, Tracheal, Esophageal, Renal and Limbs).

D. Effort is directed toward minimising complications from aspiration (suction, upright posture and prophylactic antibiotics).

E. Surgical correction via a thoracotomy, diversion of the fistula and end-to-end esophageal anastomosis.

A12.4

A. Wilms' tumour (nephroblastoma), Neuroblastomas, and liver tumour (hepatoblastoma) in order of frequency.

B. Wilms' tumour.

C. It presents between 3–4 years of age, rarely extends across the midline, is smooth on palpation and does not have X-ray calcifications. A neuroblastoma presents earlier, commonly extends across the midline, is knobby on surface palpation and has X-ray calcifications.

D. Radical surgery followed by chemotherapy provides the best chance of cure.

E. Stage and histologic subtypes; 85% of patients have favourable histology (FH); 15% have unfavourable histology (UH); overall survival is 85% for all stages.

Q12.5
This child was diagnosed with biliary atresia at birth.

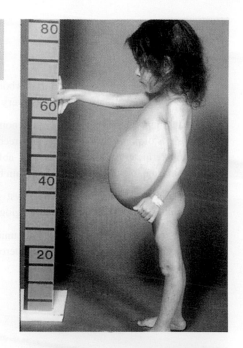

A. What is this condition? How common is it?

B. What are the signs and symptoms?

C. What investigations should be carried out?

D. Name the definitive treatment for this child's current condition.

Q12.6
A day-old female neonate was found to be passing faeces from her introitus.

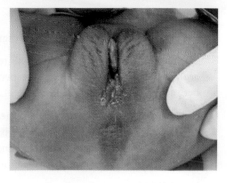

A. What is the clinical diagnosis?

B. What is the main factor that will determine how the infant's condition will be managed?

C. How can this condition be managed?

D. What are the associated anomalies?

Answers

A12.5

A. Biliary atresia is a rare condition in newborn infants in which the extrahepatic biliary ducts are blocked or absent. It occurs every one in 16,000 births.

B. Persistent jaundice, hepatomegaly, splenomegaly, ascitis, acholic stools, biliuria and other signs of portal hypertension. If unrecognised, the condition leads to liver failure but not kernicterus. The liver is still able to conjugate bilirubin and conjugated bilirubin is unable to cross the blood brain barrier.

C. Ultrasound (rule out choledochal cyst and examine extrahepatic bile ducts), cholescintigraphy (HIDA) scan, cholangiogram and liver biopsy.

D. If the intrahepatic biliary tree is unaffected, a surgical reconstruction can be performed (Kasai hepatoportoenterostomy). If atresia is complete, liver transplantation is the only option.

A12.6

A. Imperforate anus with a fistula to the vagina introitus.

B. Whether the lesion is high or low with respect to the puborectalis sling. Low lesions are characterised by a fistula to the perineum somewhere along the midline raphe between the anus the midline meatus.

C. Colostomy before reconstruction is done for high lesions. A pull-through procedure called posterior sagittal anorectoplasty is performed at a later date. Low lesions can usually be managed with immediate anoplasty or dilatation and delayed repair. A stoma is not necessary if primary repair is possible.

D. VACTERAL association. Cardiovascular anomalies occur in 15–20%

Q12.7
This is a 2-year-old boy.

A. What is your diagnosis?

B. How did this condition develop?

C. What would you expect to find upon examination?

D. How would you manage the condition?

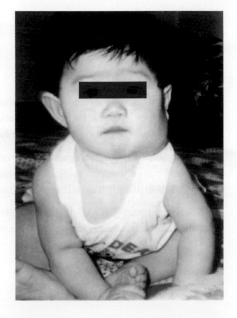

Q12.8
This is an erect X-ray of a new-born child with abdominal distension. He was suspected of having Hirchsprung's Disease.

A. Describe the two findings in the X-ray.

B. What is this disease called?

C. How do older patients of this condition present?

D. How can we confirm diagnosis?

E. What is the management?

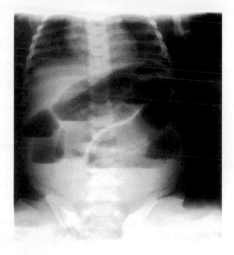

Answers

A12.7

A. Cystic hygroma.

B. At the 6th week of embryonic life, the primitive lymph sacs develop in the mesoblast, the principle pair being situated between the jugular and subclavian veins. Sequestration of a portion of the jugular lymph sacs accounts for the appearance.

C. As a result of the intercommunication of its various compartments, the swelling is soft and partially compressible, visibly increasing in size when the patient coughs or cries. It is brilliantly translucent when illuminated.

D. Sclerosant agents have been attempted. Excision of all the lymphatic bearing tissues with meticulous conservative neck dissection is the mainstay of treatment.

A12.8

A. Multiple fluid levels with distended bowel loops.

B. A congenital disorder characterised by a variable length of intestinal aganglionosis and presence of nerve hypertrophy of the hindgut.

C. They suffer chronic constipation, abdominal distension and failure to thrive.

D. A rectal suction biopsy. A full thickness specimen will allow identification of the absence of ganglion cells in the Auerbach myenteric and the Meissner submucosal plexus.

E. Initial colonic decompression to prevent enterocolitis.

   Unstable patients: diverting colostomy.

   Stable patients: reconstruction of intestinal continuity by bringing ganglionated bowel to within 1 cm of anal verge (Swenson, Duhamel and Soave procedures).

Q12.9

A 3-day-old neonate presented with bilious vomiting, abdominal distension and failure to pass meconium. The abdomen was distended with visible bowel loops.

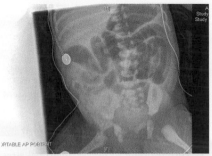

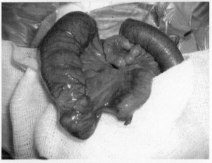

A. What is the first pathology to exclude in this clinical scenario?

B. What investigation should we perform next and why?

C. Describe the findings of the X-ray.

D. What are the possible differential diagnoses?

E. Based on the intra-operative picture, what is your diagnosis? What is the treatment?

Q12.10

A 2-year-old child had a 1-day history of abdominal pain, bilious vomiting, passing red current jelly per rectum, and a tender palpable mass in the right upper quadrant.

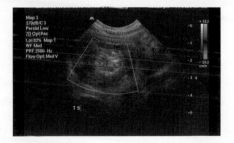

A. What was the radiological investigation performed?

B. What is your diagnosis?

C. Describe this pathological state.

D. What is the treatment for this condition?

E. What is the risk of recurrence?

Answers

A12.9

A. An imperforate anus.

B. Obtain a plain radiograph. The extent of gaseous distension of bowel suggests the level of obstruction.

C. Dilated small bowel loops, unequal sizes of bowel loops, paucity of gas in rectum.

D. Hirschsprung's Disease, intestinal atresia, meconium ileus and malrotation.

E. Intestinal atresia. Resection and primary anastomosis.

A12.10

A. Doppler ultrasound.

B. Intussusception.

C. It is the invagination of proximal bowel (intussusceptum) into the distal bowel (intussuscepien). swelling, vascular compromise and obstruction follow. It develops mostly during the first 2 years of an infant and is believed to be due to lymphoid hyperplasia in the terminal ileum after a viral infection.

D. Controlled air enema reduction is successful in 90% of cases; otherwise an operative reduction is indicated.

E. 5% from either mode of treatment.

Q12.11
A 12-year-old girl presented with a 1-day history of severe lower right-sided abdominal pain and vomiting. Menarche was at eleven. On examination, she was very tender in the right iliac fossa.

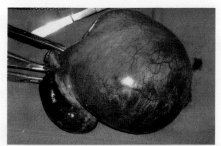

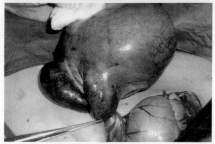

A. What are the possible differential diagnoses?

B. Which radiological investigations could be carried out to confirm your diagnoses?

C. Based on the intra-operative pictures, what is the most likely diagnosis?

Q12.12
A 15-year-old Chinese boy complained of discomfort in the right hypochondrium.

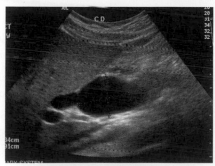

A. What can be seen in the investigations and what is the diagnosis?

B. What is this condition called?

C. How is it classified?

D. Which population group is most commonly affected?

E. What does this condition predispose the patient to?

F. How should the condition be managed?

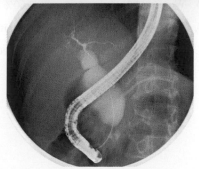

Answers

A12.11

A. Appendicitis, mesenteric adenitis, ectopic pregnancy, volvulus of a malrotated gut and torsion of the ovaries. Appendicitis is the most common acute surgical emergency.

B. Ultrasound and CT Scan.

C. Torsion of the ovary.

A12.12

A. Cystic dilatation of the common bile duct. Note the non-dilated intrahepatic biliary ducts which would be present if it were a distal obstruction. Choledochal cyst.

B. Congenital dilations of the biliary tree. They can occur in any bile duct but more characteristically in the common hepatic and common bile duct.

C. They can be classified into five types, as described by Tadoni based on the anatomical site of the cyst. This is a type 1, which is the most common whereby there is a fusiform/saccular dilatation of the CBD with normal intrahepatic ducts.

D. Women (3:1), Asian descent and 60% diagnosed before 10 years of age.

E. Jaundice, choledocholithiasis, cholangitis, portal hypertension and cholangiocarcinoma.

F. Surgical resection with biliary tree reconstruction.

Chapter **13**

NEUROSURGERY

Q13.1
A 60-year-old lady was investigated for persistent headaches.

A. What can be seen in the MRI scans?

B. Name the adverse effects of the lesion on the brain.

C. What symptoms and signs might the patient have?

D. What are the differential diagnoses of these lesions in the brain?

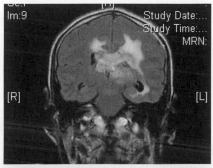

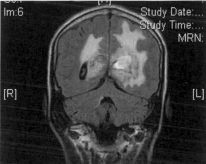

Q13.2
A 17-year-old boy was involved in a road traffic accident. Within minutes, his heart rate had dropped to 48/min.

A. What does the CT head scan show?

B. How did this condition develop?

C. What is the classical history?

D. Why is there a physiological change in his heart rate?

E. How is this treated?

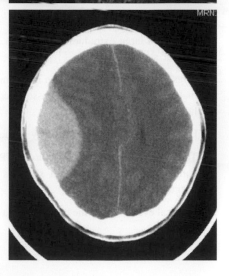

Answers

A13.1

A. A space occupying lesion/tumour in the brain.

B. The space occupying lesion causes increases intracranial pressure, mass effects on cranial nerves, invasion of brain parenchyma resulting in disruption of nuclei and tracts; seizure foci; and haemorrhage into/around the parenchyma.

C. Neurological deficit (66%), headache (50%), seizures (25%) and vomiting (classically in the morning).

D. Metastatic lesions are the most common (often originate from lung, skin, kidney, breast and colon). The primary lesions include gliomas (50%) and meningiomas (25%).

A13.2

A. There is a large extradural haematoma over the right parietal region resulting in a midline shift.

B. It results from a traumatic brain injury in which the blood builds up between the dura mater and the skull. It is often associated with a skull fracture as the bone fragments lacerate meningeal arteries.

C. Loss of consciousness followed by a "lucid interval," then neurological deterioration.

D. The expanding haematoma increases ICP, which manifests as Cushing's Reflex in the patient. The triad of clinical signs is bradycardia, hypertension and respiratory irregularity.

E. Surgical evacuation of the clot through a burr hole or craniotomy.

Q13.3
A 49-year-old lady presented with a sudden onset of headache associated with vomiting.

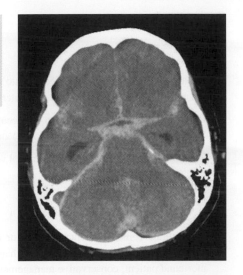

A. What does the non-contrast CT head scan show?

B. What are the common causes of this condition?

C. What kind of further investigation is appropriate?

D. What are the possible complications?

E. What are the treatment options?

Q13.4
This man had an urgent neurosurgical procedure performed.

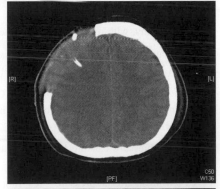

A. What had been performed on the patient?

B. Why was it necessary?

C. What is the Kellie Monroe doctrine?

D. What is cerebral perfusion pressure (CPP) and how is it derived?

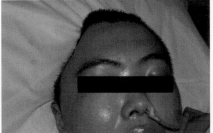

Answers

A13.3

A. Subarachnoid hemorrhage (bleeding into the subarachnoid space, which is between the arachnoid membrane and the pia mater surrounding the brain).

B. Rupture of (1) a berry aneurysm (a saccular outpouching of vessels in the circle of Willis, usually at the bifurcations) or (2) an arteriovenous malformation.

C. Cerebral four vessel angiogram (bilateral vertebral and carotid vessels).

D. 1. Brain oedema
   2. Re-bleeding
   3. Vasospasm

E. The definitive management – coiling or clipping of aneurysm. These attempts are to prevent further episode of haemorrhage, which can be life-threatening. For the moribund patient, conservative management may be appropriate.

A13.4

A. Craniectomy, with removal of part of the brain.

B. Decompression to reduce the raised intra-cranial pressure (ICP).

C. It is the pressure-volume relationship between ICP, volume of CSF, blood, brain tissue and cerebral perfusion pressure (CPP). The cranium is incompressible and the volume inside is fixed. Any increase in volume of any of its constituents will be compensated by a decrease in another.

D. It is the pressure causing blood flow to the brain. It is fairly constant due to auto-regulation.

   CPP = Mean arterial pressure – ICP (normal CPP is >70 mmHg)

Q13.5

This patient underwent a craniotomy. On the 7th post-operative day, he developed a fever and had a drop in Glasgow Coma Scale (GCS).

A. What is GCS and how is it used?

B. What are the possible causes of this condition?

C. What procedure is being performed in picture A?

D. What are the structures traversed by the spinal needle during lumbar puncture (from skin to deep)?

E. What is the normal pressure?

F. What is the procedure performed in picture B?

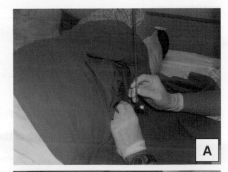

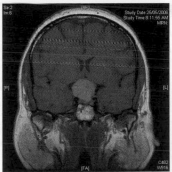

Q13.6

The 30-year-old lady suffered from persistent giddiness.

A. What can be seen in these MRI scans?

B. What is the most common type of this condition?

C. How might the patient present clinically?

D. What is the management mode?

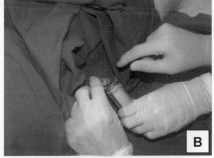

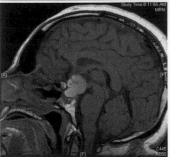

Answers

A13.5

A. Glasgow Coma Scale assesses the conscious level of the patient by using eye, speech and motor responses.

B. Post-operative meningitis or increase intracranial pressure (ICP).

C. Lumbar puncture with measurement of the ICP.

D. Skin, subcutaneous tissue, fat, supraspinous ligament, interspinous ligament, ligamentum flavum, epidural fat, dura and arachnoid into subarachnoid space.

E. Between 5 to 15 mm H_2O.

F. Collection of cerebrospinal fluid (CSF) for cytology, culture and antibiotic sensitivity.

A13.6

A. A pituitary tumour (8% of all intra-cranial tumours). They can be either classified as basophilic, acidophilic or chomophobic; based on plasma levels or immuno-histochemical staining.

B. Prolactinoma. They may be symptomatic, either from the elevated levels of prolactin in the blood or pressure effects on surrounding tissues.

C. These tumours arise from the sella turcica and can expand into the suprasellar cisterns, compressing the optic chiasma above and resulting in bilateral hemianopia (lateral fields are blind). They can cause endocrine disturbances by either hypopituitarism or excess secretion of a particular pituitary hormone.

D. Bromocriptine is used for medical treatment. Those refractory to medical treatment can undergo surgical resection via the transphenoidal route.

Chapter **14**

ORTHOPAEDICS

S Suresh Nathan

Q14.1
This 16-year-old male experienced knee pain that worsened over a 6 months period.

A. Describe the findings of the X-ray.

B. What is your diagnosis?

C. How would you stage this condition?

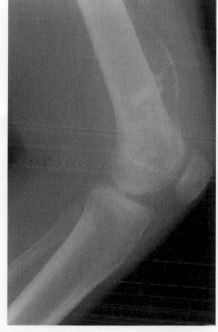

Q14.2
This 70-year-old man has a history of nasopharyngeal carcinoma.

A. What is this investigation shown in the picture?

B. What is the principle of this modality?

C. What does the investigation reveal?

D. If this condition had been found in a 19-year-old soldier, what would be your diagnosis?

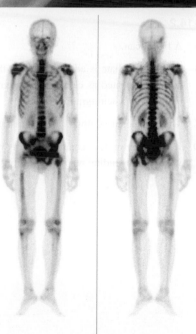

Answers

A14.1

A. Sclerotic, intraosseous, metaphyseal and permeative margins. These are all signs of an aggressive malignant process in the distal femur.

B. Osteosarcoma – in this age group, the findings are virtually diagnostic. Malignant fibrous histiocytoma of bone may develop in the elderly.

C. **Serum alkaline phosphatase**: this is a prognostic marker and reduces with good chemotherapeutic response;

   Tc99 bone scan: this delineates the tumour and shows the presence of metastatic and metacentric lesions;

   CT chest: this shows the presence of gross metastasis in the chest.

A14.2

A. A bone scan.

B. Tc-99 Phosphate is administered to the patient. It is taken up by bone-forming cells and incorporated as calcium phosphate in the bone. The radioactivity in the bone is detected by a scintigraphic camera.

C. There is increased uptake of contrast on the left hemipelvis.

D. It is clear from the scenario that this represents metastasis. In a 19-year-old soldier, a very similar finding would be seen in stress fractures.

Q14.3
This is an MRI of an Osteosarcoma in the distal femur of a 16-year-old boy.

A. Where is the epicentre of the tumour?

B. Based on the MRI, is the growth plate an effective barrier to epiphyseal spread?

C. What might preclude limb salvage surgery?

D. Is this tumour contained within the compartment of origin?

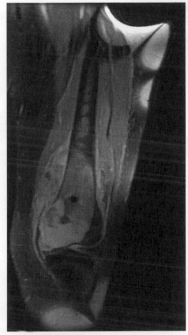

Q14.4
An 18-year-old lady complained of upper tibia pain for the past few months.

A. Describe the X-ray findings.

B. Are there other investigations required before reaching a diagnosis?

C. What is the diagnosis?

D. How should this condition be managed?

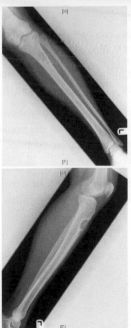

Answers

A14.3

A. Intraosseous metaphysis.

B. No. There is clear permeation of the epiphysis.

C. Incarceration of the popliteal vessel by tumour but not necessarily displacement.

D. No. Tumours that are outside their compartment of origin are prognostically worse and require wider margins of resection for cure.

A14.4

A. There is a lytic, diaphyseal, intraosseous, well-defined lesion in the upper aspect of the left tibia – these are features of a benign condition of the bone.

B. The standard for these patients are a bone scan and MRI, followed by a biopsy. A chest CT should be done in the event of suspicion of malignancy.

C. This patient had an osteofibrous dysplasia. Other differential diagnoses include non-ossifying fibroma, desmoplastic fibroma, chondromyxoid fibroma or subacute osteomyelitis. The findings are not consistent with a malignant diagnosis viz. osteosarcoma.

D. The patient should have a biopsy and curettage of the lesion and reconstruction of the defect using a bone substitute.

Q14.5
This 76-year-old man complained of bilateral knee pain, which is mechanical in nature.

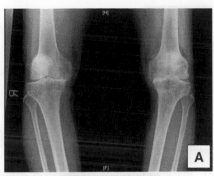

A. Describe the X-ray findings in picture A.

B. What other investigations are required to reach a diagnosis?

C. What is the diagnosis?

D. How should the condition be managed?

E. What can be seen in picture B?

F. What are the possible post-operative complications?

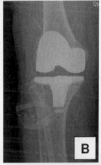

Q14.6
A 40-year-old man complained of severe pain in his left arm after a road traffic accident.

A. What is your diagnosis?

B. What is the typical mechanism of injury?

C. What are the typical physical signs?

D. What are the potential complications of this injury?

E. What are the possible treatment options?

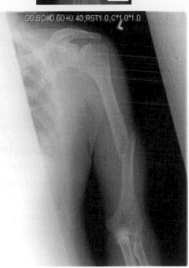

Answers

A14.5

A. Loss of joint space, subchondral sclerosis, subchondral cysts, osteophytes and varus deformity – the standard five features of osteoarthritis anywhere in the body.

B. Often none. Nevertheless, if etiology is needed, a rheumatological screen comprising rheumatoid arthritis factor, uric acid and anti-nuclear antibodies may be considered.

C. Bilateral osteoarthritis of the knee.

D. Initial treatment is conservative with analgesia, weight loss and supports. If the patient is not suitably relieved, surgery may be offered in the form of a knee joint replacement.

E. A total knee joint replacement.

F. Deep vein thrombosis, prosthetic infections and periprosthetic fractures.

A14.6

A. Left mid-shaft fracture of the humerus.

B. A fall on the outstretched arm or a direct blow.

C. Humeral shaft fractures are often rotationally unstable and can demonstrate shortening.

D. Radial nerve palsy, non-union, mal-union and delayed union.

E. **Conservative**: reduction and immobilised with a splint for 1–2 weeks, with subsequent placement in a fracture brace.

   Surgical: indicated in polytrauma, open fractures, radial nerve palsy following reduction, segmental fractures and inadequate closed reduction of failed conservative management. Options include open reduction and internal fixation (ORIF), with plate and screw or intramedullary nailing or external fixation for open fractures.

Q14.7
This patient sustained an injury to the left forearm after a fall.

A. What is the diagnosis?

B. What kind of nerve injury may be associated with this condition?

C. What is the treatment?

D. What functional disability can arise from inadequate reduction of the fracture?

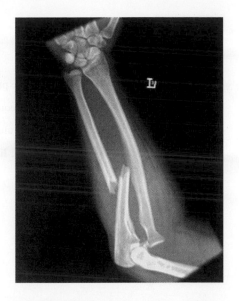

Q14.8
A 7-year-old child injured his elbow following a fall. He complained of severe pain in the forearm 2 hours later.

A. What is the radiological diagnosis in picture A?

B. What is the cause of the pain?

C. What complications may arise from this injury?

D. How can we manage the injury?

E. What kind of complication of the condition can be seen in another child, shown in picture B?

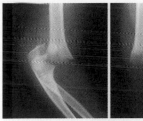

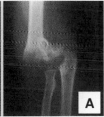

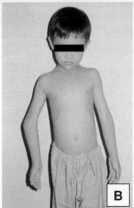

Answers

A14.7

A. Monteggia fracture-dislocation; fracture proximal ulna and dislocated radial head.

B. Radial nerve palsy or posterior interosseous nerve palsy.

C. Open reduction and internal fixation of ulna (plating) and reduction of radial head.

D. Limitation of pronation and supination; limitation of forearm rotation and limitation of elbow movement.

A14.8

A. Displaced supracondylar fracture humerus.

B. An arterial injury or compartment syndrome.

C. Volkmann's ischaemia (acute ischaemia of the muscles of the forearm), median nerve palsy, ulnar nerve palsy or brachial artery thrombosis.

D. Non-displaced: conservative management with splinting.

Displaced: percutaneous pinning and casting.

Significant swelling and neurovascular compromise require urgent reduction and close observation.

E. Cubitus varus ("Gunstock deformity") due to inadequate treatment.

Q14.9
This patient presented with a painful shoulder after sustaining an injury when playing soccer.

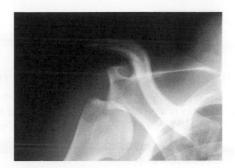

A. What is the diagnosis?

B. What pathologies or complications are associated with this injury?

C. How would you manage this patient?

Q14.10
A 70-year-old male was admitted to hospital following a fall and inability to walk.

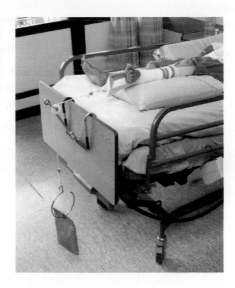

A. Name the apparatus that is used on the patient's left lower limb.

B. Why is it used?

C. Which injuries entail the need for this apparatus?

D. What are the possible complications which may arise from the use of this apparatus?

Answers

A14.9

A. Anterior dislocation of right shoulder. Over 95% of shoulder dislocation cases are anterior. Posterior dislocations are occasionally due to electrocution or seizure and may be caused by strength imbalance of the rotator cuff muscles. Inferior dislocation is the least likely form, occurring in less than 1% of all shoulder dislocation cases.

B. Hill Sach's lesion; Bankart's lesion; lax capsule and nerve injury or vascular injury.

C. Manipulation and reduction (M and R) and splintage in an arm sling.

Kocher's method is a most popular method of reducing shoulder dislocation and should be done only under anaesthesia. Traction is applied on the arm and it is abducted. It is then externally rotated and then the arm is adducted, after which it is internally rotated.

A14.10

A. Straight leg skin traction.

B. It helps to regain normal length and alignment of involved bone; reduce and immobilise a fractured bone; lessen or eliminate muscle spasms; relieve pressure on nerves and reduce/prevent skeletal deformities or muscle contractures.

C. Intertrochanteric fracture; fracture neck of femur; irritable hip; reduced dislocated hip and acetabular fracture.

D. Nerve palsy; ischaemic limb; compartment syndrome and pressure sores.

Q14.11
A 60-year-old man had low back pain and experienced occasional fever during the past 2 months.

A. What is the diagnosis?

B. How does this condition develop?

C. Which radiological features support your diagnosis?

D. What neurological deficits may occur?

E. What other investigations may be useful in confirming the diagnosis?

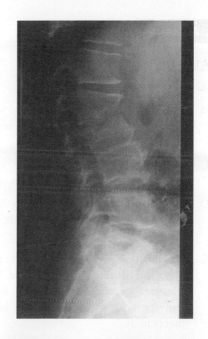

Q14.12
A 65-year-old female slipped and fell at her home. She was unable to stand.

A. What is the diagnosis, based on picture A?

B. How may this injury be classified?

C. Which underlying pathology is this injury most commonly associated with?

D. What surgery was performed in picture B?

E. What can be seen in picture C and what complications may arise after the operation?

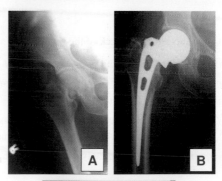

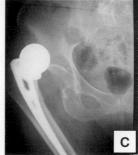

Answers

A14.11

A. Pyogenic or tuberculosis infection.

B. Pott's Disease is usually secondary to an extraspinal source of infection. It is a combination of osteomyelitis and arthritis that usually involves more than one vertebra.

C. Disc space narrowing, end plate erosion, vertebral collapse and osteopenia. Progressive bone destruction leads to vertebral collapse and kyphosis.

D. Neurologic abnormalities occur in 50% of cases and can include spinal cord compression with paraplegia, paresis, impaired sensation, nerve root pain, and/or Cauda Equina Syndrome.

E. Tuberculin skin test (purified protein derivative [PPD]) results are positive in 84–95% of patients with Pott Disease. The erythrocyte sedimentation rate (ESR) may be markedly elevated (>100 mm/h). Bone tissue or abscess samples are obtained to stain for acid-fast bacilli (AFB), and organisms are isolated for culture and susceptibility.

A14.12

A. Fracture of the neck of the right femur.

B. Garden Classification:

Type 1 is a stable fracture with impaction in valgus.

Type 2 is complete but non-displaced.

Type 3 is displaced (often rotated and angulated) with varus displacement but still has some contact between the two fragments.

Type 4 is completely displaced and there is no contact between the fracture fragments.

C. Osteoporosis.

D. Moore's Hemiarthroplasty.

E. The prosthesis has dislocated. Other complications include infection, loosening, and protusio acetabuli.

Q14.13
A 70-year-old female slipped at home and fell on the outstretched hand.

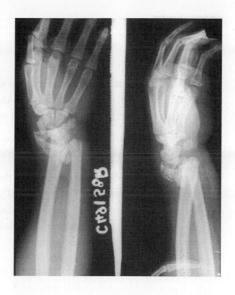

A. Describe the radiological features seen in the pictures.

B. What complications are usually associated with this kind of injury?

C. How can we manage these fractures?

Q14.14
A 12-year-old male presented with pain in the right groin after a twisting injury of the right lower limb.

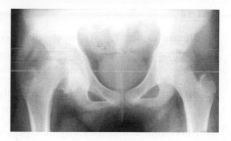

A. What is the diagnosis?

B. Which group of patients are usually affected?

C. How else do they present?

D. What can be observed during a clinical examination?

E. How do we manage this condition?

Answers

A14.13

A. Intra-articular fracture of distal radius with dorsal displacement and communition (Colles' fracture). It is named after Abraham Colles, an Irish surgeon who first described this in 1814 before the advent of X-rays.

B. Rupture of the Extensor Pollicis Longus (EPL), frozen shoulder, carpal tunnel syndrome, stiffness of the wrist, osteoarthritis and distal radio-ulnar joint instability.

C. Treatment depends on the severity of the fracture. An undisplaced fracture may be treated with a cast alone. The cast is applied with the distal fragment in ulnar deviation. A fracture with mild angulation and displacement may require closed reduction. Significant angulation and deformity may require an open reduction and internal fixation or external fixation.

A14.14

A. Slipped capital femoral epiphysis where there is a fracture/slippage through the epiphyseal growth plate. The neck comes to lie anteriorly and the head is tilted back. Cause is unclear but abnormal hormone imbalance has been hypothesised.

B. Boys in their early teens who are sexually immature for their age and in girls who are a little older and have undergone a recent growth spurt.

C. Apart from a limp, they may have pain which sometimes radiate to the knee. It may be acute or proceeded by months of discomfort.

D. There is limited abduction in flexion with loss of internal rotation.

E. Treatment is surgical. Minor/moderate: hips should be pinned in its newly deformed position. Major: gentle reduction and then pinning.

Q14.15
A 40-year-old man experienced a sudden onset of low back and left leg pain.

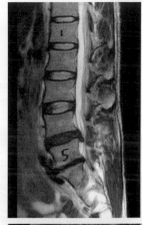
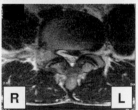

A. What scans are these and what is the diagnosis?

B. Which nerve root is most likely to be involved?

C. What is the initial management of this condition?

D. When is surgery needed?

Q14.16
This man has persistent weakness of his right hand following a laceration over the volar aspect of the wrist 3 years ago.

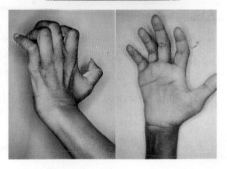

A. Which clinical features are present?

B. What is the pathophysiology?

C. What other non-traumatic causes may lead to this condition?

D. What investigation can be done to confirm the diagnosis?

Answers

A14.15

A. These are his MRI scans.

There is a left L4/5 prolapsed intervertebral disc. It is a tear in the outer, fibrous ring (annulus fibrosus) of an intervertebral disc that allows the soft, central portion (nucleus pulposus) to bulge out.

B. Left L5 nerve root.

C. Rest, analgesics and physiotherapy.

D. It is indicated if a patient has a significant neurological deficit, or if there is failure of non-surgical therapy. The presence of Cauda Equina Syndrome (incontinence, lower limb weakness and genital numbness) is considered a medical emergency requiring immediate attention and possibly surgical decompression.

A14.16

A. A claw hand and wasting of the intrinsic muscles.

B. Ulnar nerve injury.

C. Brachial plexus abnormalities, thoracic outlet syndrome, Guyon's Tunnel Syndrome, infections, tumours, diabetes, hypothyroidism, rheumatism, and alcoholism.

D. Nerve conduction test.

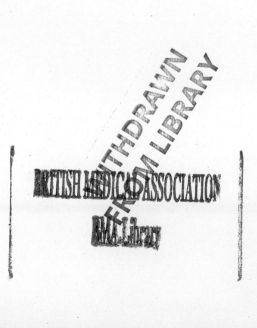